Evidence-based Clinical Chinese Medicine

Volume 4

Adult Asthma

Evidence-based Clinical Chinese Medicine

Print ISSN: 2529-7562
Online ISSN: 2529-7554

Series Co Editors-in-Chief

Charlie Changli Xue *(RMIT University, Australia)*
Chuanjian Lu *(Guangdong Provincial Hospital of Chinese Medicine, China)*

Evidence-based Clinical Chinese Medicine

Co Editors-in-Chief:

Charlie Changli Xue
RMIT University, Australia

Chuanjian Lu
Guangdong Provincial Hospital of Chinese Medicine, China

Volume 4
Adult Asthma

Lead Authors:

Johannah Shergis

Lei Wu

World Scientific

NEW JERSEY · LONDON · SINGAPORE · BEIJING · SHANGHAI · HONG KONG · TAIPEI · CHENNAI · TOKYO

Published by

World Scientific Publishing Co. Pte. Ltd.

5 Toh Tuck Link, Singapore 596224

USA office: 27 Warren Street, Suite 401-402, Hackensack, NJ 07601

UK office: 57 Shelton Street, Covent Garden, London WC2H 9HE

Library of Congress Cataloging-in-Publication Data

Names: Xue, Charlie Changli, author. | Lu, Chuan-jian, 1964– author.
Title: Evidence-based clinical Chinese medicine / Charlie Changli Xue, Chuanjian Lu.
Description: New Jersey : World Scientific, 2016. | Includes bibliographical references and index.
Identifiers: LCCN 2015030389| ISBN 9789814723084 (v. 1 : hardcover : alk. paper) |
   ISBN 9789814723091 (v. 1 : paperback : alk. paper) |
   ISBN 9789814723121 (v. 2 : hardcover : alk. paper) |
   ISBN 9789814723138 (v. 2 : paperback : alk. paper) |
   ISBN 9789814759045 (v. 3 : hardcover : alk. paper) |
   ISBN 9789814759052 (v. 3 : paperback : alk. paper)
Subjects: | MESH: Medicine, Chinese Traditional--methods. | Clinical Medicine--methods. |
   Evidence-Based Medicine--methods. | Psoriasis. | Pulmonary Disease, Chronic Obstructive.
Classification: LCC RC81 | NLM WB 55.C4 | DDC 616--dc23
LC record available at http://lccn.loc.gov/2015030389

British Library Cataloguing-in-Publication Data
A catalogue record for this book is available from the British Library.

ISBN 978-981-3203-81-5 (v. 4 : hardcover : alk. paper)
ISBN 978-981-3203-82-2 (v. 4 : paperback : alk. paper)

For any available supplementary material, please visit
http://www.worldscientific.com/worldscibooks/10.1142/9962#t=suppl

Disclaimer

The information in this monograph is based on systematic analyses of the best available evidence for Chinese medicine interventions both historical and contemporary. Every effort has been made to ensure accuracy and completeness of the data of this publication. This book is intended for clinicians, researchers, and educators. The practice of evidence-based medicine consists of considerations of the best available evidence, clinical experience and judgment of practitioners, and preferences of patients. Not all interventions are acceptable in all countries. It is important to note that some of the substances mentioned in this book may no longer be in use, may be toxic, or may be prohibited or restricted under the provisions of the Convention on International Trade in Endangered Species of Wild Fauna and Flora (CITES). Practitioners, researchers, and educators are advised to comply with the relevant regulations in their country and with the restrictions on the trade in species included in CITES appendices I, II and III. This book is not intended as a guide for self-medication. Patients should seek professional advice from their qualified Chinese medicine practitioners.

Foreword

Since the late 20th century, Chinese medicine, including acupuncture and herbal medicine, has been increasingly used throughout the world. The parallel development and spread of evidence-based medicine has provided challenges and opportunities for Chinese medicine. These opportunities include evidence-based medicine's emphasis on the effective use of the best available clinical evidence, incorporation of clinicians' clinical experience, and consideration of patients' preferences. Such practices are patient-centred, thus reflecting the historical nature of Chinese medicine practice.

However, the challenges are also significant due to the fact that, despite the long-term development of Chinese medicine and rich literature accumulated over 2,000 years, there is an overall lack of high quality clinical evidence for many of the interventions used in Chinese medicine. To address this knowledge gap, we need rigorous clinical studies to produce reliable evidence that can promote evidence-based practices of Chinese medicine.

Modern Chinese medicine is rooted in classical literature and the legacy of ancient doctors, grounded in the practice of expert modern clinicians, and increasingly informed by clinical and experimental research efforts. In recognition of the unique features of Chinese medicine, for each of the conditions in this series, a 'whole evidence' approach is used to synthesize the different types and levels of currently available evidence. This synthesis thus presents practitioners with the current best evidence and enables them to make informed clinical decisions.

There are four main components of the 'whole evidence' approach. Firstly, we present the current approaches to the diagnosis, differentiation, and treatment of each condition as suggested by textbooks and clinical guidelines. This provides an overview of how the condition is currently managed. The second section provides an analysis of the condition within a historical context based on systematic searches in the *Encyclopedia of Traditional Chinese Medicine*, which includes the full texts of more than 1,000 classical medical books. These analyses provide objective views on how the condition has been treated over two millennia, reveal continuities and discontinuities between traditional and modern practice, and suggest avenues for future research.

The third component is the assessment of evidence derived from modern clinical studies of Chinese medicine interventions. The methods established by the *Cochrane Collaboration* are used for conducting systematic reviews and performing meta-analyses of outcome data for randomised controlled trials (RCTs). In addition, the clinical relevance of data from these meta-analyses is enhanced by examining the herbal formulae, individual herbs, and acupuncture treatments that were assessed in the RCTs, and the evidence base is broadened by the inclusion of data from non-randomised, controlled clinical trials, and non-controlled studies. The fourth component is to determine how the herbal medicine interventions may achieve the effects indicated by the clinical trials. Thus, for each of the most frequently used herbs, we provide reviews of their effects in pre-clinical models and the likely underlying mechanisms of their effects.

For each condition, this 'whole evidence' approach links clinical expertise, historical precedents, clinical research data, and experimental research to provide readers with assessments of the current state of efficacy and safety for Chinese medicine interventions, including herbal medicines, acupuncture, moxibustion, and other related health care practices such as *taichi*.

Since these books are available in Chinese and English, they can benefit patients, practitioners, and educators internationally and enable practitioners to make clinical decisions informed by the current best evidence.

These publications represent a major milestone in the development of Chinese medicine and make a significant contribution to evidence-based Chinese medicine globally.

Co-Editors-in-Chief

Professor Charlie Changli Xue, RMIT University, Australia
Professor Chuanjian Lu, Guangdong Provincial
Hospital of Chinese Medicine, China

Purpose of the Monograph

This book is intended for clinicians, researchers, and educators. It can be used to inform tertiary education and clinical practice by providing systematic, multi-dimensional assessments of the best available evidence for using Chinese medicine to manage each common clinical condition.

How to use this Monograph

Definitions

A glossary is included which contains terms and definitions that frequently appear in the book. It also describes the statistical tests, methodological terms, evaluation tools, and interventions that are discussed. For example, in this book, 'integrative medicine' refers to the combined use of a Chinese medicine treatment with conventional medical management, and 'combination therapies' refer to two or more Chinese medicines from different therapy groups (Chinese herbal medicine, acupuncture, or other Chinese medicine therapies) administered together.

Data analysis and interpretation of results

In order to synthesise the clinical evidence, a range of statistical analysis approaches are used. In general, the effect size for dichotomous data is reported as a risk ratio (RR) with 95% confidence intervals (CI), and for continuous data, they are reported as mean difference (MD) with 95% CI. Statistically significant effects are indicated with an asterisk (*). Readers should note that statistical significance does not necessarily correspond with clinically important effects. Interpretation of results should also take into consideration the clinical significance of results, quality of studies (expressed as high, low, or unclear risk of bias in this book), and heterogeneity amongst the studies. Tests for heterogeneity are conducted using the I^2 statistic. An I^2 score greater than 50% is considered to indicate substantial heterogeneity.

Use of evidence in practice

The Grading of Recommendations Assessment, Development, and Evaluation (GRADE) approach was used to summarise the quality of evidence and results of the strength of evidence for critical and important comparisons and outcomes. Due to the diverse nature of Chinese medicine practice, treatment recommendations are not included with the summary of findings tables. Therefore, readers will need to interpret the evidence with reference to the local practice environment.

Limitations

Readers should note some of the methodological limitations on classical literature and clinical evidence.

- Search terms used on the *Zhong Hua Yi Dian* database may not include all terms that have been used for the condition, which may alter the findings.
- Chinese language has changed over time. Citations have been interpreted for our analysis, and such interpretations may be subject to disagreement.
- Chinese medicine theory has evolved over time. As such, concepts described in classical Chinese medical literature may no longer be found in contemporary works.

- Symptoms described in citations may be common to many conditions, and a judgment was required to determine the likelihood that the citation is related to the condition. This may have introduced some bias due to the subjective nature of the judgment.
- The vast majority of the clinical evidence for Chinese medicine treatments comes from China. The applicability of the findings to other populations and other countries requires further assessment.
- Many studies included participants with varying disease severity. Where possible, sub-group analyses were conducted to examine the effects in different sub-populations. As this was not always possible, the findings may be limited to the population included, and not to sub-populations.
- The potential risk of bias found in many included studies present methodological limitations. The findings for GRADE assessments based on studies of very low to moderate quality evidence should be interpreted accordingly.
- Nine major English and Chinese language databases were searched to identify clinical studies, in addition to clinical trial registers. Although the current search is considerably thorough, other studies may exist which were not identified, and may affect the findings.
- The calculation of frequency of herbal formulae used was based on formula names only. It is possible that studies evaluated herbal treatments with the same or similar herb ingredients, but which were given different formula names. Due to the complexity of herbal formulae, it was considered not appropriate to make a judgment as to the similarity of formulae for analysis. As such, the frequency of formulae reported in Chapter 5 may be underestimated.
- The most frequently utilised herbs that may have contributed to treatment effects have been described in Chapter 5. These herbs may provide leads for further exploration. Calculation of the herbs with potentially beneficial effects is based on frequency of formulae reported in the studies, but does not take into consideration the clinical implications and functions of every herb in a formula.

Authors and Contributors

Co-Editors-in-Chief

Prof. Charlie Changli Xue (*RMIT University, Australia*)
Prof. Chuanjian Lu (*Guangdong Provincial Hospital of Chinese Medicine, China*)

Co-Deputy Editors-in-Chief

A. Prof. Anthony Lin Zhang (*RMIT University, Australia*)
Dr. Brian H May (*RMIT University, Australia*)
Prof. Xinfeng Guo (*Guangdong Provincial Hospital of Chinese Medicine, China*)
Prof. Zehuai Wen (*Guangdong Provincial Hospital of Chinese Medicine, China*)

Lead Authors

Dr. Johannah Shergis (*RMIT University, Australia*)
Dr. Lei Wu (*Guangdong Provincial Hospital of Chinese Medicine, China*)

Co-Authors:

RMIT University (Australia):
A. Prof. Anthony Lin Zhang
Prof. Charlie Changli Xue

Guangdong Provincial Hospital of Chinese Medicine (China):

Dr. Shaonan Liu
Prof. Xinfeng Guo
Prof. Yinji Xu
Prof. Lin Lin

Members of Advisory Committee and Panel

Co-Chairs of Project Planning Committee

Prof. Peter J Coloe (*RMIT University, Australia*)
Prof. Yubo Lyu (*Guangdong Provincial Hospital of Chinese Medicine, China*)
Prof. Dacan Chen (*Guangdong Provincial Hospital of Chinese Medicine, China*)

Centre Advisory Committee (Alphabetical Order)

Prof. Keji Chen (*The Chinese Academy of Sciences, China*)
Prof. Aiping Lu (*Hong Kong Baptist University, China*)
Prof. Caroline Smith (*University of Western Sydney, Australia*)
Prof. David F Story (*RMIT University, Australia*)

Methodology Expert Advisory Panel (Alphabetical Order)

Prof. Zhaoxiang Bian (*Hong Kong Baptist University, China*)
The late Prof. George Lewith (*University of Southampton, United Kingdom*)
Prof. Jianping Liu (*Beijing University of Chinese Medicine, China*)
Prof. Frank Thien (*Monash University, Australia*)
Prof. Jialiang Wang (*Sichuan University, China*)

Content Expert Advisory Panel (Alphabetical Order)

Prof. Jingcheng Dong (*Institute of Integrative Medicine of Fudan University, China*)
Prof. Frank Thien (*Monash University, Australia*)
Dr. Christopher Worsnop (*Austin Health, Australia*)

Professor Charlie Changli Xue, PhD

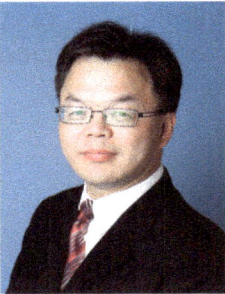

Professor Charlie Changli Xue holds a Bachelor of Medicine (majoring in Chinese Medicine) from Guangzhou University of Chinese Medicine, China (1987), and a PhD from RMIT University, Australia (2000). He has been an academic, researcher, regulator, and practitioner for almost three decades. Prof. Xue has made significant contributions to evidence-based educational development, clinical research, regulatory framework and policy development, and provision of high quality clinical care to the community. Prof. Xue is recognised internationally as an expert in evidence-based traditional medicine and integrative health care.

Prof. Xue is the Inaugural National Chair of the Chinese Medicine Board of Australia appointed by the Australian Health Workforce Ministerial Council (in 2011), and he was reappointed for the second term in 2014. Since 2007, he has been a Member of the World Health Organization (WHO) Expert Advisory Panel for Traditional and Complementary Medicine, Geneva. Prof. Xue is also Honorary Senior Principal Research Fellow at the Guangdong Provincial Academy of Chinese Medical Sciences, China.

At RMIT, Prof. Xue serves as the Executive Dean for the School of Health and Biomedical Sciences. He is also the Director of the WHO Collaborating Centre for Traditional Medicine.

Between 1995 and 2010, Prof. Xue was Discipline Head of Chinese Medicine at RMIT University. He leads the development of five successful undergraduate and postgraduate degree programmes in Chinese Medicine at RMIT University, which is now a global leader in Chinese medicine education and research.

Prof. Xue's research has been supported by research grants worth over AU$15 million, including six project grants from the Australian Government's National Health and Medical Research Council (NHMRC) and two grants from the Australian Research Council (ARC). He has contributed over 200 publications and has been frequently invited as a keynote speaker for numerous national and international conferences. Prof. Xue has contributed to over 300 media interviews on issues related to complementary medicine education, research, regulation, and practice.

Professor Chuanjian Lu, MD

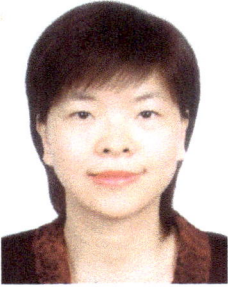

Professor Chuanjian Lu holds a Doctor of Medicine from Guangzhou University of Traditional Chinese Medicine. She is the Vice President of Guangdong Provincial Hospital of Chinese Medicine (Guangdong Provincial Academy of Chinese Medical Sciences, Second Clinical Medical College of Guangzhou University of Chinese Medicine). She also is the Chair of the Guangdong Traditional Chinese Medicine (TCM) Standardization Technical Committee, and the Vice-chair of the Immunity Specialty Committee of the World Federation of Chinese Medicine Societies (WFCMS).

Prof. Lu has engaged in scientific research on TCM, clinical practice, and teaching for some 25 years. She has devoted her research to integrated traditional and Western medicine and has edited and published 12 monographs and 120 academic research articles as first author and corresponding author, with over 30 articles being included in Science Citation Index journals.

Prof. Lu has received widespread recognition for her achievements with awards including the 'Excellent Teacher of South China,' 'National Outstanding Women TCM Doctor,' and 'National Outstanding Young Doctor of TCM.' She also received 'The Science and Technology Star of the Association of Chinese Medicine,' the 'National Excellent Science and Technology Workers of China Award,' and the 'Five-Continent Women's Scientific Awards of China Medical Women's Association.'

Prof. Lu has also won the 'Award of Science and Technology Progress' conferred by the Guangdong Provincial Government, China Association of Chinese Medicine, and Chinese Hospital Association over 10 times.

Acknowledgments

The authors and contributors would like to acknowledge the valuable contributions of research assistants and students who provided assistance for the electronic database search and screening for the evaluation of clinical evidence. We also acknowledge the assistance of Dr. Neil Owens in editing the manuscript.

Contents

List of Figures

List of Tables

1

Introduction to Asthma

OVERVIEW

Asthma is a significant worldwide health problem. The prevalence of asthma is increasing and asthma currently affects an estimated 300 million people. Poorly controlled asthma undermines one's quality of life and can also be fatal. Asthma can be chronic or acutely worsen when exacerbated. Symptoms, which include wheezing, shortness of breath, chest tightness, and cough, can be persistent or intermittent and may be triggered by one or more stimuli such as allergens, exercise, or cold air. Asthmatics are encouraged to avoid triggers but symptoms may also require treatment. The goal of treatment is to manage and control symptoms and reduce exacerbations. However, there is currently no cure for asthma. Children and adults with asthma are often managed differently and treatment protocols vary between these groups. This monograph evaluates Chinese medicine for adult asthma, focusing on individuals over the age of 18. This chapter describes the definition, risk factors, pathological processes, diagnosis and management of adult asthma based on internationally recognised conventional medicine guidelines.

Definition of Asthma

The cause of asthma is not fully understood, but research indicates that it is a combination of genetic predisposition and exposure to environmental triggers. Asthma is often allergy-induced and children with allergies may experience more variable symptoms whereas adults often experience more persistent symptoms. People who develop asthma as adults may not have reacted to allergens as a child, but over time their body starts to respond differently. The underlying mechanisms of adult and childhood asthma are very similar, but most research focuses on either group to address their individual needs and management strategies.

Asthma causes inflammation in the airways leading to airway hyperresponsiveness to environmental triggers. Common triggers are viruses, house dust mites, pollen, dust, exercise, animal dander, and cold air. Clinically, asthma is defined by reversible airways obstruction, with episodes of shortness of breath, wheezing, chest tightness, and coughing. Variability in symptoms and airflow obstruction is typical. The airflow obstruction is caused by inflammation with mucosal oedema, epithelial desquamation, and increased mucus secretion, as well as contraction of airway smooth muscle. Remodelling of the airways causes muscle layer and basement membrane thickening and fibrosis in the airway wall. Asthma symptoms may be prominent at night or in the early morning and vary from day-to-day.[1]

Prevalence

Asthma is a significant health and economic problem globally. Asthma affects over 300 million people worldwide and accounts for approximately 1% of the total global burden of disease.[2] Asthma rates have been increasing since the 1980s,[3] influenced by several factors including increased awareness, changes in diagnosis, and a shift towards an urban lifestyle.

The prevalence of asthma varies between countries, ranging from 1% to 18%.[2] The prevalence is higher in western counties, such as the USA, UK, and Australia, and lower in Asian countries, such as China.[4]

Risk Factors

Genetics, family history, and environmental factors contribute to the risk of a person developing asthma. Emerging evidence shows that, for susceptible people, the development of the immune system in the early years of life plays a significant role in altering the risk of developing asthma.[1] Predisposing genetic factors from a number of familial genes can make an individual susceptible to atopy and airway hyper-responsiveness. These individuals are more likely to develop asthma and are vulnerable to sensitisation by otherwise innocuous triggers such as allergens (e.g., pollen, pet dander, dust mites, and mould), infections, tobacco smoke, exercise, weather conditions, occupational irritants, and air pollution. Asthma primarily develops in childhood and may spontaneously resolve in early adulthood. Some adults, although previously unaffected by asthma, may develop symptoms later in life. Occupational triggers may be the cause; however in most cases the reason is not known.

Tobacco smoking, including passive smoking, can contribute to the development of asthma and lead to more severe symptoms, lung function decline, and reduction of drug effectiveness.[5] *In utero* and neonatal smoke exposure is associated with higher chance of developing cough, wheezing, and shortness of breath in the first few years of life.[6]

Other risk factors for asthma are obesity and male sex.[7] Boys are two times more likely to develop childhood asthma than girls. However, observations in the adult population show that the prevalence evens and becomes similar between the sexes, and in some cases slightly higher in women than men.

Pathological Processes

Inflammation of the airways is the key feature of asthma. The inflammatory process is complex and involves many cells, such as eosinophils, T lymphocytes, mast cells, and macrophages.[3] Exposure to environmental factors such as allergens and infections leads to asthma symptoms and morphological changes. In non-asthmatics the stimulating environmental factors do not cause a response, yet in asthmatics these 'innocuous' influences cause airway hyperresponsiveness. A multi-faceted and abnormally amplified immune response ensues and leads to physiological effects throughout the airway. After many exposures, the airways undergo an inflammation and repair cycle, which can lead to permanent damage.[1]

During an acute episode of asthma, airway smooth muscle contracts, inflammatory cells migrate, and oedema thickens the airway walls. If previous sensitisation has occurred, the response is likely to be over-exaggerated and worsened by existing structural changes. Triggering factors stimulate inflammatory cells and airway epithelial cells to release a variety of inflammatory mediators (e.g., chemokines and cytokines), which mediate inflammation and attract additional inflammatory cells. The cytokines (e.g., interleukin (IL) -1β and tumour necrosis factor alpha (TNF-α)) coordinate the inflammation and type 2 T helper cells (Th2; e.g., IL-4, IL-5, and IL-13) promote eosinophil differentiation and immunoglobulin E (IgE) formation. Other mediators such as histamine from mast cells cause constriction of the bronchi and promote inflammation.

After multiple acute episodes, airways undergo narrowing due to structural changes such as laying-down of collagen beneath the epithelium, known as fibrosis.[9] Smooth muscle cells also increase in size and number and blood vessels proliferate causing swelling of the airway walls.[9] Mucus is increased as submucosal glands become larger and greater numbers of goblet cells migrate to the airways.

Diagnosis

The diagnosis of asthma is based on the combination of typical symptoms, such as shortness of breath, coughing, wheezing, and tightness of the chest, and the demonstration of airflow obstruction that is variably reversible or fully reversible.[1] Asthma is a chronic disease and symptoms can acutely worsen (especially at night) after exposure to triggers, such as pollen, smoke, and infections. The existence of a family history of asthma and other allergic diseases may also contribute to patient diagnosis.[1]

Diagnostic Assessment

Physical examination may show no signs of abnormality. Sometimes wheeze can be heard, but other conditions can also cause wheeze. The typical symptoms, shortness of breath and wheezing, may be present in some patients but not in all. Spirometry is used to demonstrate airway obstruction to confirm a diagnosis. Lung function is measured by forced expiratory volume in one second (FEV$_1$), forced vital capacity (FVC), and peak expiratory flow (PEF). Airflow obstruction is defined as the FEV$_1$/FVC ratio being less than the lower limit in the normal range. Spirometry is often performed pre- and post-administration of a short-acting bronchodilator. If the FEV$_1$ or FVC improves by more than 12% and 200 mL, then the bronchodilator has had a real effect of dilating the airways. The larger the improvement, the more likely asthma is the appropriate diagnosis. If the prebronchodilator results show obstruction and the post-administration results are normal, this indicates an asthma diagnosis especially when other signs and symptoms are present. However, the 12% change may not always be diagnostic of asthma because approximately half of patients with chronic obstructive pulmonary disease (COPD) will have a significant acute bronchodilator response and some patients with asthma may not have a response. Overall, the asthma diagnosis is based on the clinical picture in combination with demonstration of airflow obstruction.

For people with normal spirometry at the time of testing, an asthma challenge test will help to determine the diagnosis. A peak flow reading in isolation is not used to diagnose asthma because it has poor sensitivity and specificity. Peak flow readings over time can be helpful for monitoring asthma. Other measures, such as inflammation in the airways measured by sputum eosinophils and neutrophils may guide treatment but are not diagnostic. Exhaled nitric oxide levels may also assist with treatment, but are not sensitive enough to use for diagnosis and are generally not available.[10] Challenge testing with known allergic triggers can be used to confirm aggravating factors.

Ongoing assessment of patients with asthma is important and symptom control is the goal of management. Asthma control is defined as: 1) no daytime symptoms, 2) no limitation of daily activities, including exercise, 3) no night-time symptoms or waking due to asthma, 4) no need for reliever treatment, and 5) normal or near-normal lung function. Partially controlled asthma includes daytime symptoms more than twice per week, limitation of activities, night-time symptoms, reliever treatment more than twice per week, and lung function as assessed by PEF or FEV_1, < 80%. People with uncontrolled asthma experience three or more features of partially controlled asthma.[1]

Differential Diagnosis

Conditions such as cough-variant asthma, angiotensin converting enzyme (ACE) induced cough, and eosinophilic bronchitis should be considered. Cough-variant asthma is identified in patients with a primary symptom of chronic cough. The cough is worse at night and daytime cough may be absent. ACE-induced cough has a clear history of medication use, and eosinophilic bronchitis presents with cough, increased sputum eosinophils but normal lung function, and no hyperresponsiveness of the airway.

Other conditions such as COPD, parenchymal lung disease, and left ventricular failure, sometimes known as cardiac asthma, need to be differentiated from asthma. In adults, asthma may be difficult to distinguish from COPD and at times they will both be present. Asthma usually responds well to treatment over time, whereas COPD has irreversible airflow obstruction even with optimal treatments. Left ventricular failure can be distinguished from asthma using chest x-ray, and electrocardiography (ECG) and high-resolution computed tomography (HRCT) scans can also be used to diagnose parenchymal lung disease.

Vocal cord dysfunction can sometimes be confused with asthma, or they may co-exist giving a false impression that asthma is not well controlled. Obesity can be associated with dyspnoea, cough, and wheeze without airway disease. Therefore, the assessment of airflow obstruction is important in diagnosing asthma.

Other Diagnostic Considerations

Up to 30% of people with rhinitis have asthma. Rhinosinusitis often shares risk factors with asthma, potentially contributing to exacerbations and increasing the severity of asthma.[1] Gastroesophageal reflux is also common in asthma patients and can cause cough.[11] A proper differential diagnosis needs to be conducted to ensure gastroesophageal reflux is not contributing to asthma symptoms. Up to 28% of adults with asthma and taking aspirin or nonsteroidal anti-inflammatory drugs may experience exacerbated asthma symptoms.[12]

Acute Exacerbations of Asthma

Exacerbations are characterised by acute worsening of cough, wheeze, shortness of breath, chest tightness, and lung function. Exacerbations put patients at risk of respiratory distress, hypoxemia, and airflow obstruction, and serve as the most important marker of asthma management and treatment effectiveness.[13] In some cases, the patient may require hospitalisation. Triggers of exacerbation may include viral respiratory tract infections, allergens (e.g., pet dander, pollen, and mould), tobacco smoke, exercise, weather conditions, occupational irritants, and air pollution. In some cases, the trigger is unknown.

Management

The primary objectives of asthma management are to control symptoms, maintain lung function and activity levels, and prevent asthma exacerbations and mortality. Optimal treatment early in the course of the disease can improve patient outcomes. Treatments should aim to stabilise symptoms for long periods and prevent exacerbation.[1] To objectively measure asthma over time, questionnaires include the Asthma Control Test (ACT), Asthma Therapy Assessment Questionnaire, and the Asthma Quality of Life Questionnaire (AQLQ). Regular monitoring of peak flows and spirometry is also recommended.

Pharmacological Treatments

Treatments for asthma are categorised as relievers or controllers (Table 1.1).[1] Relievers are used on an as-needed basis when symptoms flare up, giving quick relief. They include bronchodilators such

Table 1.1   Treatment Recommendations for Asthma

Options	Step 1 Reliever Medication	Step 2 Reliever Medication Plus a Controller	Step 3 Reliever Medication Plus One or Two Controllers	Step 4 Reliever Medication Plus Two or More Controllers	Step 5 Reliever Medication Plus Additional Controllers
Recommended	As-needed short-acting beta2-agonists	Low-dose ICS	Low-dose ICS plus LABAs	Medium-High dose ICS plus LABAs	Oral glucocorticosteroids
Alternative		Leukotriene modifier	Medium-High dose LABAs or Low-dose ICS plus leukotriene modifier or Low-dose ICS plus theophylline	Leukotriene modifier or Theophylline	Anti-IgE treatment

Table adapted from GINA 2013.[1]

Abbreviations: ICS, inhaled corticosteroid; LABA, long-acting beta2-agonist.

as β_2-adrenoceptor agonists (beta2-agonists) and anticholinergics. Controllers are used daily for long periods to stabilise asthma symptoms. Controllers reduce airway inflammation and include glucocorticosteroids, long acting beta2-agonists, leukotriene antagonists, theophylline, and anti-IgE-monoclonal antibodies.

Controller medications are stepped-up when asthma symptoms become uncontrolled and stepped-down when asthma becomes controlled (Table 1.1). Most asthma medications are inhaled. This administration system allows the medication to be delivered directly to the airways, producing concentrated effects and reducing side effects.[1]

Reliever Medications

Inhaled short-acting beta2-agonists (SABAs) are the recommended bronchodilators for rapid relief of asthma symptoms, including salbutamol and terbutaline.[1] Known adverse side effects include tremor and tachycardia.[1] Anticholinergics, such as inhaled ipratropium, tiotropium, and oxitropium, are used to relieve asthma symptoms but they are not as effective as SABAs. Anticholinergics can be used by patients experiencing side effects from SABAs. Systemic corticosteroids can also be used in severe cases of asthma exacerbations. They do not provide immediate relief but can be used for five to 10 days to reduce the severity of exacerbations.[1] Theophylline may also have some positive effects for relieving acute asthma symptoms but they are not first-line treatments.[1]

Controller Medications

International guidelines recommend inhaled glucocorticosteroids as the main controller medication (Table 1.1). Inhaled corticosteroids (ICS) include budesonide, fluticasone proprionate, fluticasone furorate, ciclesonide, and beclomethasone. Research shows they reduce symptoms and asthma exacerbations, suppress inflammation, and improve overall lung function and quality of life.[14,15] However, long-term use can also produce undesirable side effects such as increased fracture risk, oropharyngeal candidiasis, bruising, and osteoporosis.[16] In addition, cessation of ICS after long-term use can cause symptom relapse and increased airway inflammation. Thus, while systemic glucocorticosteroids can be used in selected patients if ICS do not control symptoms, long-term use is not recommended due to side effects.

Long-acting beta2-agonists (LABAs) combined with ICS are used as controller medications for asthma. The combination of ICS and LABAs produces better control of asthma and can be given at lower doses than ICS alone. Fixed dose combinations are used and these include fluticasone proprionate/salmeterol, budesonide/formoterol and mometasone/formoterol, fluticasone propriante/formoterol, and fluticasone furorate/vilanterol. Fixed combinations of budesonide/formoterol are effective as controller and reliever medication[17] and side effects of LABAs are reportedly few.[18]

Other controller medications include leukotriene modifiers such as montelukast, zafirlukast, and pranlukast. They can reduce cough and airway inflammation while improving lung function, yet their effects are inferior to ICS. Leukotriene modifiers can help reduce the dose of ICS and enhance asthma control.[1] While theophylline, which is an anti-inflammatory bronchodilator, is not commonly prescribed for first-line controller treatment, combining theophylline with ICS can help control symptoms better in some patients. Side effects of theophylline are common and include arrhythmias, convulsions, headaches, insomnia, nausea, and gastrointestinal upset. Anti-IgE including the monoclonal antibody, omalizumab, is given to patients with high levels of serum IgE and can reduce asthma exacerbations and hospitalisations.[19] Although anti-IgE is rarely used, it plays an important a role in treating patients with severe allergic asthma and those with uncontrolled symptoms despite ICS and oral prednisolone. While side effects are rare, however, Churg-strauss syndrome has been reported in patients coming off ICS aided by IgE therapy.[20]

Other Medications

Selected asthma patients with an identified trigger may benefit from immunotherapy. Tolerance to allergens is the goal of therapy, and successful therapy can effectively reduce symptoms and medication use.[21] However, the effects of current immunotherapies are small compared with other controller medications such as ICS, and side effects such as anaphylaxis and asthma exacerbations have been reported.[21]

Non-pharmacological Interventions

Asthma patients also use non-pharmacological interventions such as breathing techniques, smoking cessation, exercise, diet therapy, and vaccination. However, the effectiveness of these interventions has not been well established. Self-management, education, and emergency plans for acute exacerbations are proven to reduce morbidity.[1] Teaching patients to understand, monitor, and manage their own asthma can enable patients to make pre-planned changes to medications based on how well their symptoms are controlled.

Prognosis

Asthma is not curable, yet effective and holistic management can control symptoms and prevent deterioration of lung function. Triggers such as allergens or indoor and outdoor pollution should be avoided where possible and occupational exposure should be removed. If asthmatics smoke, their symptoms will be difficult to treat and their lungs will be impaired. Therefore, smoking cessation should be a high priority for people with asthma. Asthmatics are encouraged to develop an action plan with their health care provider, which should include education and medication awareness that aims to give them control over their condition. If the guided self-management plans are properly developed and implemented, asthma morbidity will be greatly reduced.[1] A chapter summary is presented in Table 1.2.

Table 1.2   Chapter Summary

Definition of asthma	• Inflammation in the airways leads to airway hyperresponsiveness. • Reversible airways obstruction, with episodes of shortness of breath, wheezing, chest tightness, and coughing.
Diagnosis	• Patient history of symptoms including shortness of breath, wheezing, chest tightness, and coughing. • Reversible airflow obstruction. • History of symptoms triggered by viruses, house dust mites, pollens, dusts, exercise and animal dander.
Non-pharmacological management	• Avoid triggers • Develop an asthma action plan • Smoking cessation
Pharmacological management	• Inhaled bronchodilators (short-acting, long-acting) • Inhaled corticosteroids • Combination of inhaled bronchodilators and corticosteroids

References

1. Global Strategy for Asthma Management and Prevention. Global Initiative for Asthma (GINA). Updated 2015. Available from: http://www.ginasthma.org/.

2. Masoli M, Fabian D, Holt S, Beasley R. The global burden of asthma: executive summary of the GINA Dissemination Committee report. Allergy. 2004;**59**(5):469–78.

3. Akinbami L, Moorman J, Liu X. Asthma Prevalence, Health Care Use, and Mortality: United States, 2005–2009. Number 32. U.S. Department of Health and Human Services. Centers for Disease Control and Prevention. National Center for Health Statistics. 2011.

4. Asher MI, Montefort S, Bjorksten B, Lai CK, Strachan DP, Weiland SK, *et al*. Worldwide time trends in the prevalence of symptoms of asthma, allergic rhinoconjunctivitis, and eczema in childhood: ISAAC Phases One and Three repeat multicountry cross-sectional surveys. Lancet. 2006;**368**(9537):733–43.

5. Thomson NC, Chaudhuri R, Livingston E. Asthma and cigarette smoking. Eur Respir J. 2004;**24**(5):822–33.

6. Ferrante G, Antona R, Malizia V, Montalbano L, Corsello G, Grutta SL. Smoke exposure as a risk factor for asthma in childhood: A review of current evidence. Allergy Asthma Proc. 2014;**35**(6):482–8.

7. Rasmussen F, Hancox RJ. Mechanisms of obesity in asthma. Curr Opin Allergy Clin Immunol. 2014;**14**(1):35–43.

8. Busse WW, Lemanske Jr RF. Asthma. NEJM. 2001;**344**(5):350–62.

9. Bergeron C, Boulet LP. Structural changes in airway diseases: Characteristics, mechanisms, consequences, and pharmacologic modulation. Chest. 2006;**129**(4):1068–87.

10. Smith AD, Cowan JO, Brassett KP, Herbison GP, Taylor DR. Use of exhaled nitric oxide measurements to guide treatment in chronic asthma. NEJM. 2005;**352**(21):2163–73+258.

11. Kiljander TO, Harding SM, Field SK, Stein MR, Nelson HS, Ekelund J, *et al.* Effects of esomeprazole 40 mg twice daily on asthma: A randomized placebo-controlled trial. Am J Respir Crit Care Med. 2006; **173**(10):1091–7.

12. Szczeklik A, Stevenson DD. Aspirin-induced asthma: Advances in pathogenesis, diagnosis, and management. J Allergy Clin Immunol. 2003;**111**(5):913–21.

13. Reddel HK, Taylor DR, Bateman ED, Boulet LP, Boushey HA, Busse WW, *et al.* An official American Thoracic Society/European Respiratory Society statement: asthma control and exacerbations: Standardizing endpoints for clinical asthma trials and clinical practice. Am J Respir Crit Care Med. 2009;**180**(1):59–99.

14. Juniper EF, Kline PA, Vanzieleghem MA, Ramsdale EH, O'Byrne PM, Hargreave FE. Effect of long-term treatment with an inhaled corticosteroid (budesonide) on airway hyperresponsiveness and clinical asthma in nonsteroid-dependent asthmatics. Am J Respir Crit Care Med. 1990; **142**(4):832–6.

15. Jeffery PK, Godfrey RW, Adelroth E, Nelson F, Rogers A, Johansson SA. Effects of treatment on airway inflammation and thickening of basement membrane reticular collagen in asthma. A quantitative light and electron microscopic study. Am J Respir Crit Care Med. 1992; **145**(4 Pt 1):890–9.

16. Passalacqua G, Albano M, Canonica GW, Bachert C, Van Cauwenberge P, Davies RJ, *et al.* Inhaled and nasal corticosteroids: Safety aspects. Allergy: Eur J Allergy Clin Immunol. 2000;**55**(1):16–33.

17. Rabe KF, Pizzichini E, Stallberg B, Romero S, Balanzat AM, Atienza T, *et al.* Budesonide/formoterol in a single inhaler for maintenance and

relief in mild-to-moderate asthma: A randomized, double-blind trial. Chest. 2006;**129**(2):246–56.

18. Jaeschke R, O'Byrne PM, Mejza F, Nair P, Lesniak W, Brozek J, *et al*. The safety of long-acting beta-agonists among patients with asthma using inhaled corticosteroids: Systematic review and metaanalysis. Am J Respir Crit Care Med. 2008;**178**(10):1009–16.

19. Normansell R, Walker S, Milan SJ, Walters EH, Nair P. Omalizumab for asthma in adults and children. Cochrane Database Syst Rev. 2014;1:Cd003559.

20. Wechsler ME, Wong DA, Miller MK, Lawrence-Miyasaki L. Churg-strauss syndrome in patients treated with omalizumab. Chest. 2009;**136**(2):507–18.

21. Abramson MJ, Puy RM, Weiner JM. Allergen immunotherapy for asthma. Cochrane Database Syst Rev. 2003;(4):Cd001186.

2

Asthma in Chinese Medicine

OVERVIEW

This chapter describes the main Chinese medicine syndromes for both stable and acute exacerbations of asthma. Treatments are taken from clinical texts and practice guidelines and include Chinese herbal medicine, acupuncture, and other non-medical therapies such as *tai chi* 太极 and *qigong* 气功.

Introduction

Asthma is known as *xiao bing* 哮病 (wheezing disease) or *xiao zheng* 哮证 (wheezing syndrome) in Chinese medicine (CM).[1] Asthma patients often face a combination of pathogenic attacks with underlying meridian deficiencies, and the common syndromes include Lung, Spleen, and Kidney meridian deficiency and phlegm. Pathogens such as cold, heat, and wind can trigger asthma exacerbations and impede the ability of the Lungs to disperse and descend *qi*. Characteristic symptoms include wheezing, breathlessness, chest tightness, coughing, and excess sputum production.[2]

Aetiology and Pathogenesis

Asthma is often caused by a combination of an excess of pathogens and deficiencies. There is persistent sputum in the Lung which increases the susceptibility of patients to external pathogenic attacks from cold and heat. Acute exacerbations may also be caused by improper diet, excess emotions, weather changes, exercise, fatigue, or stress. Phlegm blocks the airway, impairing the dispersing and descending function of the Lungs, leading to shortness of breath and wheezing.[1,2]

Asthma affects the Lung, Spleen, and Kidney meridians. Lung dominates *qi* and controls dispersing and descending. If external pathogens or pathogenic *qi* attack the Lungs, they will fail to disperse and descend *qi,* and *qi* will adversely ascend causing shortness of breath and wheezing. The Lung governs *qi* and Kidney is the root of *qi*. If wheezing persists, the Lung will become deficient and impede Kidney function. This will lead to impaired reception of *qi* and the patient's condition will become aggravated.[2]

Phlegm, the main pathological factor in asthma, is caused by improper diets and affects the Spleen's ability to transport and transform essence and nutrition (i.e., water and food). Sputum is subsequently produced and stored in the Lungs, which further aggravates symptoms. Phlegm is also related to external pathogenic factors and dysfunction of the Spleen and Kidney (Figure 2.1).[3] If cold is a factor

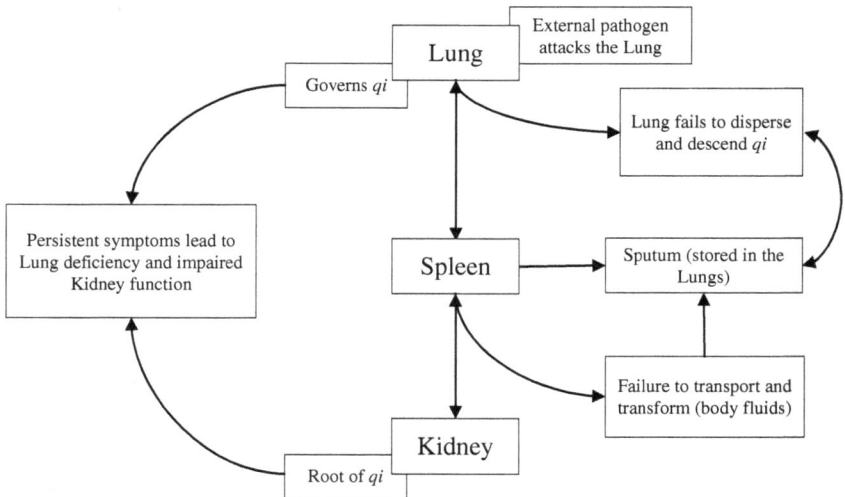

Figure 2.1. Pathogenesis of asthma in Chinese medicine.

and there is an underlying *yang* deficiency, the phlegm will become cold-phlegm and lead to cold wheezing. If heat is a factor and there is an underlying exuberance of *yang*, phlegm will become heat-phlegm and lead to heat wheezing. When phlegm is retained and wind invades, turbid phlegm will obstruct the Lung causing excess Lung *qi* (*fei qi yong shi* 肺气壅实) and wind wheezing. Deficiency of the Lungs and Spleen, retention of phlegm in the Lung, and impairment of dispersing and descending functions will lead to phlegm wheezing. If there are many acute attacks or persistent symptoms, vital *qi* will be consumed, causing Lung and Kidney deficiency and weak wheezing.[1,2]

The Lung, Spleen, and Kidney are connected in the pathogenesis of asthma. Healthy Lungs purify and send the inhaled air to the Spleen to produce *qi*. The Lungs also support the Spleen to regulate fluid. The Kidney is the root of *qi* and receives *qi* from the Lungs. In people with asthma, the Lungs fail to disperse and descend *qi* due to external pathogenic factors and/or phlegm. If the Spleen is dysfunctional, body fluids will transform into sputum which is stored in the Lung. When symptoms are chronic, Kidney *qi* is consumed, weakening the constitution.

Syndrome Differentiation and Treatments

Treatment of asthma includes reducing excess pathogens at the acute stage and strengthening the roots at the stable stage.[1,2,4] During acute exacerbations, pathogens should be identified and cold and heat should be differentiated. If there is an exterior syndrome, it should be treated by releasing the exterior. Cold-phlegm should be treated by warming and ventilating the Lung. Heat-phlegm should be treated by clearing heat from the Lungs. Wind-phlegm should be treated by expelling wind and resolving phlegm. If patients have repeated attacks which cause the deficiency of healthy *qi* and lead to an exuberance of pathogenic factors, deficiency should be tonified and reduced the excess of pathogens. If *qi* is not reinforced, wheezing and dyspnoea may worsen, leading to respiratory arrest in severe cases. During stable asthma, the main pathogenesis is the deficiency of healthy *qi* and phlegm fluid retention. Stable asthma can be treated by supporting the *yin* and *yang* roots. *Yang qi* deficiency is treated by warming and tonifying while *yin* deficiency is treated by nourishing *yin*. Meanwhile, tonifying the Lung, invigorating the Spleen, and nourishing the Kidney will help to alleviate, reduce, and control exacerbations. The pathogenesis of asthma includes deficiency of healthy *qi* and excess pathogenic *qi* caused by turbid phlegm, which obstructs the Lung and hinders the dispersing and descending functions.

CM treatments include Chinese herbal medicine (CHM), acupuncture, and other therapies such as *tuina* 推拿, *qigong* 气功, and cupping. CM treatments can be integrated with conventional medicine. Asthma is a complicated pathogenic condition and treatment should be based on its clinical manifestations and stage. Tonifying deficiency and firming the root are treatments used during chronic stable asthma to reduce excess during acute exacerbations. CM can also ventilate the Lung, improve constitution, regulate immune function, prevent pathogenic attacks, and improve quality of life.[4]

CM treatments recommended by guidelines, expert consensus, textbooks, and monographs are referred to in this section (Table 2.1). References include the Chinese Medicine Diseases Clinical Guideline for Common Diseases in Traditional Chinese Medicine Internal Medicine; Guideline on Traditional Chinese Medicine Clinical Treatments–Features and Advantages; Expert Consensus of Chinese Medicine Diagnosis and Treatment of Asthma (2012); Internal Medicine of Chinese Medicine; and Practical Internal Medicine of Chinese Medicine.[1–5] The formulae listed are referenced to the *Zhong Yi Fang Ji Da Ci Dian* 中医方剂大辞典 (ZYFJDCD), with citation numbers following the formula.[6] Note that the use of some herbs such as *ma huang* 麻黄 may be restricted in some countries. In addition, some herbs such as *chen xiang* 沉香 and *jing da ji* 京大戟 are listed under the provisions of Convention on International Trade in Endangered Species of Wild Fauna and Hora (CITES). Readers are advised to comply with relevant regulations.

Table 2.1   Summary of CHM for Asthma

Stage	Syndrome Differentiation	Treatment Principle	Formula
Chronic asthma	Lung-Spleen *qi* deficiency	Invigorate the Spleen and tonify Lung	Liu jun zi tang, modified 六君子汤
	Lung-Kidney deficiency	Tonify Lung and Kidney	Bu fei san plus Jin shui Liu Jun Jian 补肺散, 合金水六君煎
Acute exacerbations of asthma (acute stage)	Cold wheezing	Dispel cold	She gan ma huang tang, modified 射干麻黄汤
	Heat wheezing	Clear heat	Ma xing shi gan tang, modified 麻杏石甘汤
	Wind wheezing	Disperse wind	Huang long shu chuan tang 黄龙舒喘汤
	Phlegm wheezing	Resolve phlegm	San zi yang qin tang, modified 三子养亲汤
	Weak wheezing	Tonify Lung and Kidney	Ping chuan gu ben tang 平喘固本汤
	Wheezing collapse	Tonify Lung and Kidney, restore *yang*	Hui yang ji jiu tang 回阳急救汤

Chinese Herbal Medicine Treatment Based on Syndrome Differentiation

Chronic Asthma (Stable Stage)

Chronic asthma manifests as deficiency of the Lung, Spleen, and/or Kidney and symptoms are chronic and recurring. This section focuses on the two main syndromes for stable asthma, that is, Lung-Spleen *qi* deficiency and Lung-Kidney deficiency.

Lung-Spleen Qi Deficiency

<u>Clinical manifestations:</u> Shortness of breath, low voice, excessive white and thin phlegm, spontaneous sweating, aversion to wind, high susceptibility to cold, listlessness, reduced appetite, loose

stools, pale tongue, white tongue coating, thready and weak pulse, or soggy pulse.

<u>Treatment principle:</u> Invigorate the Spleen and tonify the Lung.

<u>Formula:</u> Modified *Liu jun zi tang* 六君子汤 (ZYFJDCD no. 17964).

<u>Herbs:</u> *Dang shen* 党参, *bai zhu* 白术, *fu ling* 茯苓, *shan yao* 山药, *yi yi ren* 薏苡仁, *fa ban xia* 法半夏, *chen pi* 陈皮, *wu wei zi* 五味子, *gan cao* 甘草.

<u>Analysis of formula:</u> *Dang shen, bai zhu, fu ling, shan yao,* and *yi yi ren* invigorate the Spleen and tonify *qi. Fa ban xia* and *chen pi* dry dampness and resolve phlegm. *Wu wei zi* astringes the Lung. *Gan cao* harmonises the formula.

<u>Manufactured medicines:</u> *Liu jun zi wan* 六君子丸,[3] *Zi sheng wan* 资生丸,[3] *Yu ping feng san* 玉屏风散.[4]

Lung-Kidney Deficiency

<u>Clinical manifestations:</u> Shortness of breath, rapid breathing (tachypnoea) especially after activity, difficult inspiration, thick frothy sputum, soreness and weakness of the waist and knees, vertigo and tinnitus, fatigue, vexing heat in the chest, palms, and soles, red complexion especially on the cheeks, thirst, red tongue, scanty tongue coat, thready and rapid pulse, aversion to cold, cold limbs, pale complexion, pale and enlarged tongue, white tongue coating, or deep and thready pulse.

<u>Treatment principle:</u> Tonify the Lung and Kidney.

<u>Formula:</u> *Bu fei san* 补肺散 (ZYFJDCD no. 45317) and *Jin shui liu jun jian* 合金水六君煎 (ZYFJDCD no. 52394).

<u>Herbs:</u> *Sang bai pi* 桑白皮, *shu di huang* 熟地黄, *ren shen* 人参, *zi wan* 紫菀, *wu wei zi* 五味子, *dang gui* 当归, *fa ban xia* 法半夏, *chen pi* 陈皮, *fu ling* 茯苓, *gan cao* 甘草.

<u>Analysis of formula:</u> *Shu di huang* tonifies the Kidney and improves *qi* reception. *Ren shen* and *wu wei zi* tonify *qi* and nourish the *yin* of

the Lung. *Fu ling* invigorates the Spleen and replenishes *qi*. *Fa ban xia* and *chen pi* regulate *qi* and resolve phlegm. *Sang bai pi* and *zi wan* relieve cough and resolve sputum. *Dang gui* tonifies *qi* and activates Blood. *Gan cao* harmonises the formula.

<u>Manufactured medicines:</u> *Jin gui shen qi wan* 金匮肾气丸,[3] and *He che da zao wan* 河车大造丸.[2]

Single Herb Formula

1. *Di long* 地龙: Dry and grind into powder. Consume 3g twice per day. Suitable for heat wheezing.[5]
2. *Zao jiao* 皂角: Decoct 15g and add 30g of *bai jie zi* 白芥子 12 hours later. Dry and grind into powder. Consume 1-1.5g three times per day. Suitable for phlegm wheezing.[5]

Acute Exacerbations of Asthma (Acute Stage)

Acute stage asthma can manifest as an excess of pathogens or deficient syndrome, and can be due to cold, heat, wind, or phlegm. Acute stage asthma may also be classified as weak wheezing or wheezing collapse. These syndromes are classified as the acute stage because they occur acutely with significant worsening of symptoms that may lead to collapse and respiratory arrest. The underlying causes are deficient Lung and Kidney *qi* and *yang* that are worsened by excess pathogenic factors.

Cold Wheezing

<u>Clinical manifestations:</u> Dyspnoea, tachypnoea, audible wheezing, fullness and stuffiness of the chest and diaphragm, scanty white frothy sputum that is difficult to expectorate, absence of thirst or thirsty for hot drinks, aversion to cold, asthma symptoms appear after catching a cold, green grey complexion, white and slippery tongue coating, wiry and tight pulse, or floating and tight pulse.

<u>Treatment principle:</u> Ventilate the Lung, dispel cold, resolve phlegm, and relieve dyspnoea.

<u>Formula:</u> Modified *She gan ma huang tang* 射干麻黄汤 (ZYFJDCD no. 70665).

<u>Herbs:</u> *She gan* 射干, *zhi ma huang* 炙麻黄, *sheng jiang* 生姜, *xi xin* 细辛, *zi wan* 紫菀, *kuan dong hua* 款冬花, *zi su zi* 紫苏子.

<u>Analysis of formula:</u> *She gan* and *zhi ma huang* ventilate the Lung, relieve dyspnoea, resolve phlegm and relieve dysfunction of the throat. *Sheng jiang* and *xi xin* warm the Lung and resolve fluid retention. *Zi wan* and *kuan dong hua* resolve phlegm and reduce coughing. *Zi su zi* descends *qi* and relieves dyspnoea.

Heat Wheezing

<u>Clinical manifestations:</u> Dyspnoea, tachypnoea, audible wheezing, fullness in the chest and hypochondrium, bouts of irritating cough, yellow or white phlegm, thick phlegm that is difficult to expectorate, heavy thirst and desire to drink, bitter taste in the mouth, sweating, red complexion or fever, external pathogen attack in the summer, red tongue, yellow greasy tongue coating, slippery and rapid pulse, or wiry and slippery pulse.

<u>Treatment principle:</u> Clear heat and ventilate the Lung, resolve phlegm, and relieve dyspnoea.

<u>Formula:</u> Modified *Ma xing shi gan tang* 麻杏石甘汤 (ZYFJDCD no. 80337).

<u>Herbs:</u> *Zhi ma huang* 炙麻黄, *xing ren* 杏仁, *shi gao* 石膏, *gan cao* 甘草, *sang bai pi* 桑白皮, *kuan dong hua* 款冬花, *fa ban xia* 法半夏, *bai guo* 白果, *huang qin* 黄芩.

<u>Analysis of formula:</u> *Zhi ma huang* ventilates the Lung and relieves dyspnoea. *Shi gao* restricts warming property of *ma huang*. *Huang qin* and *sang bai pi* clear heat and Lung. *Xing ren*, *ban xia* and *kuan dong hua* resolve phlegm and downbear counterflow. *Bai guo* astringes the Lung and relieves dyspnoea. *Gan cao* harmonises the formula.

Wind Wheezing

<u>Clinical manifestations:</u> Dyspnoea, tachypnoea, noisy breathing, cough, thick phlegm that is difficult to expectorate, no obvious cold or heat, onset and remission is usually rapid, itchy nose, throat, eyes or ears before onset, sneezing, nasal obstruction, running nose, white thin tongue coating, wiry pulse.

<u>Treatment principle:</u> Disperse wind, ventilate the Lung, and relieve dyspnoea.

<u>Formula:</u> *Huang long shu chuan tang* 黄龙舒喘汤.[1]

<u>Herbs:</u> *Zhi ma huang* 炙麻黄, *di long* 地黄, *chan tui* 蝉蜕, *zi su zi* 紫苏子, *shi chang pu* 石菖蒲, *bai shao* 白芍, *bai guo* 白果, *gan cao* 甘草, *fang feng* 防风.

<u>Analysis of formula:</u> *Zhi ma huang* ventilates the Lung and relieves dyspnoea. *Di long* extinguishes wind and relieves asthma. *Zi su zi* descends *qi* and improves dyspnoea. *Chan tui, fang feng,* and *bai shao* relieve asthma. *Bai guo* astringes the Lung and relieves dyspnoea. *Gan cao* harmonises the formula.

Phlegm Wheezing

<u>Clinical manifestations:</u> Dyspnoea, tightness in the chest, gurgling in the throat, wood-sawing sounds in the throat, orthopnoea, excessive phlegm that is easy to expectorate, green grey complexion, thick or yellow greasy tongue coating, or slippery and full pulse.

<u>Treatment principle:</u> Invigorate the Spleen and resolve phlegm, descend *qi* and relieve dyspnoea.

<u>Formula:</u> Modified *San zi yang qin tang* 三子养亲汤 (ZYFJDCD no. 5011).

<u>Herbs:</u> *Bai jie zi* 白芥子, *su zi* 苏子, *lai fu zi* 莱菔子, *zhi ma huang* 炙麻黄, *xing ren* 杏仁, *ju hong* 橘红, *fa ban xia* 法半夏, *fu ling* 茯苓, *he zi* 诃子, *gan cao* 甘草.

<u>Analysis of formula:</u> *Zhi ma huang, xing ren*, and *su zi* relieve cough and dyspnoea. *Bai jie zi, lai fu zi, ju hong*, and *fa ban xia* resolve sputum. *Fu ling* invigorates the Spleen. *He zi* astringes the Lung. *Gan cao* harmonises the formula.

Weak Wheezing

<u>Clinical manifestations:</u> Shortness of breath, exertional dyspnoea, frequent onset, possible continuous wheezing, low voice, cyanosis of lips, fingers and toes, weak expectoration, thick frothy phlegm or thin sputum, red complexion especially on the cheeks, pale complexion, dry throat with or without thirst, vexing heat, aversion to cold, cold limbs, red or dark purple tongue, pale tongue, thready and rapid pulse, or deep and thready pulse.

<u>Treatment principle:</u> Tonify Lung and Kidney, descend *qi*, and relieve dyspnoea.

<u>Formula:</u> *Ping chuan gu ben tang* 平喘固本汤.[1]

<u>Herbs:</u> *Dang shen* 党参, *wu wei zi* 五味子, *dong chong xia cao* 冬虫夏草, *hu tao rou* 胡桃肉, *chen xiang* 沉香, *ci shi* 磁石, *su zi* 苏子, *kuan dong hua* 款冬花, *fa ban xia* 法半夏, *ju hong* 橘红.

<u>Analysis of formula:</u> *Dang shen* tonifies Lung *qi*. *Hu tao rou, chen xiang, dong chong xia cao*, and *wu wei zi* nourish Kidney to receive *qi*. *Ci shi* improves *qi* reception and relieves dyspnoea. *Su zi, fa ban xia, kuan dong hua*, and *ju hong* descend *qi* and resolves phlegm.

Wheezing Collapse

<u>Clinical manifestations:</u> Repeated attacks of wheezing, audible wheezing, visible efforts to breathe with nasal flaring, open mouth and raised shoulders, shortness of breath, dysphoria, mental confusion, cyanotic complexion, cold limbs, oily sweat, green grey tongue, greasy or slippery tongue coating, thready and rapid pulse, or floating pulse without root.

<u>Treatment principle:</u> Tonify Lung and Kidney, and restore *yang* to stop collapse.

<u>Formula:</u> *Hui yang ji jiu tang* 回阳急救汤 (ZYFJDCD no. 33708).

<u>Herbs:</u> *fu zi* 附子, *gan jiang* 干姜, *rou gui* 肉桂, *ren shen* 人参, *bai zhu* 白术, *fu ling* 茯苓, *chen pi* 陈皮, *gan cao* 甘草, *wu wei zi* 五味子.

<u>Analysis of formula:</u> *Ren shen, fu zi, gan jiang,* and *rou gui* warm the interior of the body and restore *yang* and pulse. *Bai zhu, fu ling,* and *chen pi* invigorate the Spleen and resolve phlegm. *Wu wei zi* is an astringent to stop collapse. *Gan cao* harmonises the formula.

Acupuncture Therapies and Other Chinese Medicine Therapies

Acupuncture points are selected according to syndrome differentiation. Typical acupuncture points include:[1,3,5]

Chronic Asthma (Stable Stage)

- GV14 *Dazhui* 大椎 — tonifies *qi* and *yang*
- BL13 *Feishu* 肺俞 — tonifies Lung *qi*
- ST36 *Zusanli* 足三里 — tonifies the middle and benefits *qi*
- CV22 *Tiantu* 天突 — descends *qi* and resolves Phlegm
- BL23 *Shenshu* 肾俞 — tonifies Kidney and consolidates the body

Acute Exacerbations of Asthma (Acute Stage)

- EX-B1 *Dingchuan* 定喘 — stops dyspnoea
- CV22 *Tiantu* 天突 — descends *qi* and resolves Phlegm
- PC6 *Neiguan* 内关 — regulates chest *qi* and stops dyspnoea
- BL12 *Fengmen* 风门 — opens the Lungs and stops coughing and dyspnoea
- CV17 *Danzhong* 膻中 — regulates *qi*, opens the chest, and stops coughing and dyspnoea
- ST40 *Fenglong* 丰隆 — invigorates the Spleen and resolves Phlegm

In the acute stage, it is recommended that acupuncture should be administered with strong stimulation (rotated every 5–10 minutes) and needles should be retained for 30 minutes. Treatments may be given every day or every second day, with 10 days per treatment period. During the stable stage, acupuncture should be administered with mild stimulation and treatment should be done every two days. Moxibustion can also be used on the above points daily with 10 days per treatment period.

Other Management Strategies

- Depending on physical condition, people with asthma should engage in physical exercise, such as *tai chi* 太极 and *qigong* 气功 (e.g. *ba duan jin* 八段锦, eight-sectioned brocade style), to strengthen physique and improve disease resistance.[1,2]
- Asthma triggers should be identified and avoided. Patients should pay attention to air circulation of bedrooms and ensure suitable temperature and humidity. Irritant gas, dust, and pollen should be avoided. Diet should be light and nourishing, and raw, cold, fatty, and spicy foods as well as seafood should be avoided. Patients should abstain from tobacco and alcohol. They should keep warm to prevent catching a cold, avoid unhealthy or exuberant emotions, and avoid overwork and tiredness.[1,2]

References

1. 晁恩祥, 孙增涛, 刘恩顺. 支气管哮喘中医诊疗专家共识 (2012). 中医杂志. 2013 (07):627–629.
2. 吴勉华, 王新月. 全国中医药行业高等教育"十二五"规划教材, 中医内科学. 北京:中国中医药出版社, 2013.
3. 王永炎. 严世芸. 实用中医内科学. 第2版. 上海: 上海科学技术出版社. 2009.
4. 罗云坚. 孙塑伦. 中医临床治疗特色与优势指南. 北京: 人民卫生出版社. 2007.

5. 中华中医药学会. 中医内科常见病诊疗指南 中医疾病部分. 北京: 中国中医药出版社. 2008.

6. Peng HR, ed. 彭怀仁. 中医方剂大辞典. 北京:人民卫生出版社. 1997.

3

Classical Chinese Medicine Literature

OVERVIEW

Classical Chinese medicine texts are a fundamental source of information for Chinese medicine theory and practice. These ancient books include descriptions of asthma or asthma-like symptoms and treatments. This chapter includes findings from a search of the *Zhong Hua Yi Dian* 中华医典, one of the largest collections of classical Chinese medicine texts. Terms for wheeze, asthma, and abnormal breathing sounds were searched and over 1,000 citations were analysed. Formulae, herbs, and acupuncture points used in ancient Chinese medicinal practice are identified along with important quotations and citations.

Introduction

Throughout the history of Chinese medicine (CM), the understanding of asthma has undergone multiple developments and can be traced by the evolution of terms used to describe it. Before the Song Dynasty, the main terms that are used for asthma in modern times, *xiao bing* 哮病 (wheezing disease) and *xiao zheng* 哮证 (wheezing syndrome), were never mentioned. However, there were descriptions of similar symptoms. The first description of asthma appeared in the *Huangdi Neijing* 黄帝内经, or *Yellow Emperor's Classic of Internal Medicine* (c. 220 AD). The text describes various types of dyspnoea and sputum, including *chuan ming* 喘鸣, *chuan hu* 喘呼, and *chuan he* 喘喝. The *Jin Gui Yao Lue* 金匮要略, also published during the Han Dynasty, described symptoms of asthma attacks, including cough, abnormal rising of *qi*, and audible wheezing.[1] In another book, *Zhou Hou Bei Ji Fang* 肘后备急方, published in 363 AD, asthma was described as as *shang qi ming xi* 上气鸣息 (abnormal rising of *qi* and wheezing) and *xia ya xi qi* 呷呀息气 (dyspnoea and sputum).[2] During the Sui Dynasty (581–618 AD), asthma symptoms were described as *xia sou* 呷嗽 (cough with sputum and gurgling in the throat).[3] During the Tang Dynasty (618–960 AD), the terminology once again changed and books such as *Bei Ji Qian Jin Yao Fang* 备急千金要方 and *Qian Jin Yi Fang* 千金翼方 described sputum as *shui ji sheng* 水鸡声 (wheezing sounds) and *chui guan sheng* 吹管声 (breathing with a pipe-blowing sound),[4,5] and the *Wai Tai Mi Yao* 外台秘要 described asthma as *hou li ya sheng* 喉里呀声 (raspy sound in the throat).[6]

It wasn't until the Song Dynasty (961–1271) that the modern terms for asthma began to appear. The book *Zhen Jiu Zi Sheng Jing* 针灸资生经 (c. 1220) used the term *xiao chuan* 哮喘 (asthma)[7] and the book *Yi Shuo* 医说 (c. 1224) referred to asthma as *hou chuan* 齁喘 (dyspnoea and sputum).[8] *Zhu Dan Xi* 朱丹溪 further elaborated on the term *xiao chuan* in *Dan Xi Xin Fa* 丹溪心法, which was published during the Yuan Dynasty in 1481.[9] This book also mentioned both the differences and relationship between *xiao bing* 哮病 (wheezing disease) and *chuan bing* 喘病 (dyspnoea).[10] During the Ming Dynasty (1369–1644) and Qing Dynasty (1645–1911), asthma terms such as *xiao* 哮, *hou he* 齁鉿 (dyspnoea and sputum in children), *hou xia* 齁齁 (dyspnoea and sputum in children), *hou sou* 齁嗽 (wheezing with cough), and *hou ji* 齁疾 (wheezing) were further discussed in books such as *Yi Xue Zheng Zhuan* 医学正传, *Zheng Zhi Zhun Sheng* 证治准绳, and *Pu Ji Fang* 普济方.[11–13] Syndrome differentiation was mentioned much later in the Qing Dynasty in books such as *Lei Zheng Zhi Cai* 类证治裁, and terms included *leng xiao* 冷哮 (Cold wheezing), *re xiao* 热哮 (Heat wheezing), *yan xiao* 盐哮 (Salty wheezing), *jiu xiao* 酒哮 (Alcohol wheezing), and *tang xiao* 糖哮 (Sugar wheezing).[14]

Classical Literature Search

Classical literature is the foundation that guides the practice of CM. Modern books still reference information from traditional sources and clinical practice has been enriched by classical knowledge. Asthma is commonly referenced in classical literature and includes symptoms such as wheezing, dyspnoea, cough, chest tightness, and phlegm.

To obtain a sample of the classical and pre-modern medical literature, we conducted electronic searches of the *Zhong Hua Yi Dian* 中华医典 (ZHYD), or *Encyclopaedia of Traditional Chinese Medicine*, which comprised of more than 1,000 medical books.[15] This represents the largest collection currently available and is also representative of other large collections of classical and pre-modern CM literature.[16,17]

Search Procedure and Data Coding

Each search term was entered into the ZHYD search field and the search results were downloaded into spread sheets. A 'citation' was defined as a distinct passage of text referring to one or more of the search terms. Codes were allocated for types of citations, books, and the dynasties in which they were written according to the procedures described in May *et al.* 2014.[17] Books written after 1949 were excluded. Search terms included *xiao* 哮 (wheezing), *shang qi* and *shui ji* 上气+水鸡 (abnormal rising of *qi* and wheezing sounds), *chuan hu* 喘呼 (dyspnoea with laboured breathing), *chuan ming* 喘鸣 (dyspnoea and wheezing), *hou chuan* 齁喘 (dyspnoea and sputum), *chuan he* 喘喝 (dyspnoea with laboured breathing), *hou ji* 齁疾 (wheezing disease), *chui guan sheng* 吹管声 (breathing with a pipe-blowing sound), *xia ya xi qi* 呷呀息气 (dyspnoea and sputum), *shang qi ming xi* 上气鸣息 (abnormal rising of *qi* and wheezing), *hou li ya sheng* 喉里呀声 (raspy sound in the throat), and *hou sou* 齁嗽 (cough and sonorous wheeze).

Data Analysis Procedure

The number of hits identified by each search term was calculated by summing the results of the searches. After removing duplicates, exclusion criteria were then applied to remove citations which were considered unrelated to asthma. Citations which contained insufficient or no information to judge the relevance of the source to asthma were also excluded.

All relevant citations were reviewed to identify the best descriptions of asthma. Relevant citations which did not include treatment were excluded from further analysis. The final data set thus included citations considered to refer to asthma and which described CM treatments (i.e., Chinese herbal medicine (CHM), acupuncture, or other CM therapies). When a citation referred to multiple treatments, each treatment was considered as a separate citation for calculation of formulae, herbs, or acupuncture points. Citations which were pharmacopeia-type entries were reviewed for eligibility. Pharmacopeia entries which mentioned the name of the condition but did not include either a detailed description of the condition or information about treatment were excluded from further analysis. Pharmacopeia entries which included a description of the condition, with or without reference to other herbs, were included. Single acupuncture points were reviewed in a similar manner.

Included citations were grouped according to the CM intervention for further analysis. An additional screening process was performed to identify citations considered 'most likely' to be describing asthma. Results include the frequencies of herbal formulae, herbs, and acupuncture points described in these citations.

Search Results

Over 1,000 classical literature citations make a reference to respiratory symptoms including wheezing, dyspnoea, cough, chest tightness, and phlegm (Figure 3.1). Citations were also found in over 100 books written between 206 and 1949. Experts in asthma and classical literature coded the citations to indicate if they described one or more of the common asthma symptoms (e.g., wheezing, dyspnoea, cough, chest tightness, and sputum). Citations were also coded for paroxysmal attacks, worsening of symptoms at night or in the morning, triggers such as exercise, cold air, food, catching a cold, and the conditions of adults, children, infants, or post-partum women. After

Search	The Encyclopaedia of Traditional Chinese Medicine which contains over 1,000 books
Collect	Collect citations that mention any of the search terms (Table 3.1)
Sort	Sort citations and remove those that are not relevant
Analyse	Identify formulae, herbs, and acupuncture points

Total citations = 1,109
Asthma citations = 971

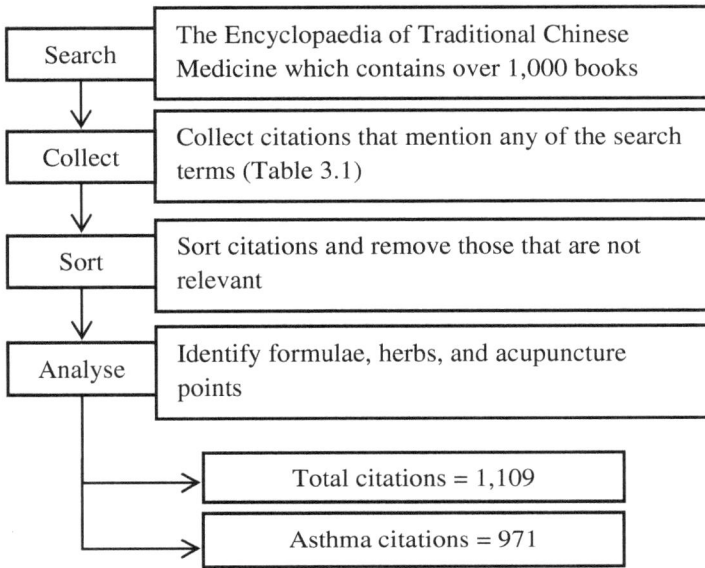

Figure 3.1. Classical literature citations.

the citations were coded, those that were found to be inconsistent with asthma were excluded from the final analysis. Excluded citations included those that described respiratory infections, cardiac diseases, and post-partum conditions, to name a few.

A total of 1,109 citations described respiratory symptoms such as cough, dyspnoea, and phlegm retention in the lungs. A total of 971 citations described asthma or a condition that is consistent with asthma. CHM was used in 869 citations, acupuncture in 93 citations, other CM therapies in six, and a combination of CHM and acupuncture in three citations.

Search Terms

The definition and terminology of asthma has undergone several changes over time and there is no direct correspondence between modern and classical terms. In order to find classical literature citations, individual symptoms of asthma were searched and two main

Table 3.1   Frequency of Search Terms

Search Term	Possible Meaning of the Term	Citations Frequency n (%)
Xiao 哮	Wheezing	685 (70.5%)
Shang qi + shui ji 上气+水鸡	Abnormal rising of qi and wheezing sounds	147 (15.1%)
Chuan hu 喘呼	Dyspnoea with laboured breathing	41 (4.2%)
Chuan ming 喘鸣	Dyspnoea and wheezing	35 (3.6%)
Hou chuan 齁喘	Dyspnoea and sputum	33 (3.4%)
Chuan he 喘喝	Dyspnoea with laboured breathing	18 (1.9%)
Hou ji 齁疾	Wheezing disease	5 (0.5%)
Chui guan sheng 吹管声	Breathing with a pipe-blowing sound	3 (0.3%)
Xia ya xi qi 呷呀息气	Dyspnoea and sputum	2 (0.2%)
Shang qi ming xi 上气鸣息	Abnormal rising of qi and wheezing	1 (0.1%)
Hou li ya sheng 喉里呀声	Raspy sound in the throat	1 (0.1%)
Hou sou 齁嗽	Cough and sonorous wheeze	0 (0%)

categories, dyspnoea and wheezing, were included. Twelve search terms were used to identify asthma citations (Table 3.1). The search focused on adults and typical patterns of asthma; therefore, the terms which describe children and individual symptoms of cough were not evaluated. Evaluation of all 971 asthma citations showed that *xiao* 哮 (wheeze) was found in most citations (685, 70.5%), followed by abnormal rising of *qi* and wheezing sounds, *shang qi* 上气 and *shui ji* 水鸡 (147, 15.1%). *Xiao* 哮 first appeared in *Zhen Jiu Jia Yi Jing* 针灸甲乙经 (c. 259) and was used in all dynasties up until today. This shows that *xiao* 哮 has been consistently used to describe asthma in ancient Chinese literature.

The other terms for wheezing are *chuan ming* 喘鸣 and *hou ji* 齁疾, which located 35 (3.6%) and five (0.5%) citations, respectively. The dyspnoea terms *chuan he* 喘喝, *chuan hu* 喘呼, and *hou chuan*

齁喘 located 92 citations (9.4%). This small number is due to the broad definition of these terms that encompass asthma as well as many other respiratory conditions, and many of the citations referred to wheezing and dyspnoea but did not provide enough information to be sure that they referred to asthma. *Hou sou* 齁嗽 did not locate any asthma citations.

Terms for wheezing, dyspnoea, and abnormal breathing sounds (*chui guan sheng* 吹管声, *hou li ya sheng* 喉里呀声, *xia ya xi qi* 呷呀息气, and *shang qi ming xi* 上气鸣息) only located seven citations (0.7%). These terms referred to cough with upward rising of *qi* but did not describe asthma. When the terms *shang qi* 上气 and *shui ji* 水鸡 were searched together, 147 citations were found (15.1%). Most described asthma with abnormal rising of *qi* and wheezing or cough.

Frequency of Citations by Dynasty

Citations were published in books spanning all the Chinese dynasties from before the Tang Dynasty (c. 618) up to and including the Ming Guo period, or the Republic of China (1912–1949) (Table 3.2). Citations published in modern China after 1949 were not included in the results. The earliest citation was from the *Shang Han Lun* 伤寒论 (Han Dynasty; c. 206). Between the Han and Yuan Dynasties, only a few citations were found (8.7%). During and after the Ming Dynasty (1369–1644), book publishing expanded and fundamental CM texts like the first official medical encyclopaedia, the *Sheng Ji Zong Lu* 圣济总录, or *Collected Prescriptions for Divine Relief from Suffering*, were published, as was the famous *Ben Cao Gang Mu* 本草纲目. This expansion of book publishing is likely the reason for most of the citations (85.5%) being found in books written during the Ming and Qing Dynasties. Books published during the Ming Guo or Republic of China period made up a small number (5.8%) of the sampled works, because the Ming Guo period spanned only 37 years (1912–1949) compared to the Ming and Qing Dynasties that spanned over 500 years.

Table 3.2 Search Term by Dynasty

Dynasty		Search Terms										
	Xiao 哮	Shang qi + shui ji 上气+水鸡	Chuan ming 喘鸣	Chuan hu 喘呼	Chuan he 喘喝	Hou chuan 齁喘	Hou ji 齁疾	Chui guan sheng 吹管声	Xia ya xi qi 呷呀嗽气	Shang qi ming xi 上气鸣息	Hou li ya sheng 喉里呀声	Hou sou 齁嗽
Before Tang Dynasty (before 618)	1	4	1	1	1	0	0	0	1	0	0	0
Tang and 5 Dynasties (618–960)	1	17	2	0	1	0	0	2	0	1	0	0
Song and Jin Dynasties (961–1271)	4	27	6	1	3	0	0	0	0	0	0	0
Yuan Dynasty (1272–1368)	7	2	0	0	2	0	0	0	0	0	0	0
Ming Dynasty (1369–1644)	164	38	6	17	8	16	5	1	1	0	1	0
Qing Dynasty (1645–1911)	466	55	16	16	3	17	0	0	0	0	0	0
Ming Guo/Republic of China (1912–1949)	42	4	4	6	0	0	0	0	0	0	0	0
Total	685	147	35	41	18	33	5	3	2	1	1	0

Asthma Symptoms

Each classical literature citation referred to wheezing and dyspnoea except for one that described phlegm-type chronic asthma. Chest tightness was only described in six citations. Cough accompanied wheezing and dyspnoea in 299 citations (31%) and sputum production was described in 314 citations (32.3%). Forty-one citations (4.2%) mentioned that symptoms were worse at night or in the early morning, and 44 (4.5%) described paroxysmal attacks.

Wheezing, dyspnoea, and cough were triggered by cold air in 169 citations (17.4%). Food was a trigger in 40 citations (4.1%) and external pathogenic attack leading to asthma symptoms was mentioned in 13 citations (1.3%); the remaining citations did not mention the aetiology of asthma. Symptoms were described as chronic in 119 citations (12.3%).

Patient case reports accounted for 134 of the citations (13.8%). The book *Xu Min Yi Lei An* 续名医类案, written by Wei Zhixiu 魏之琇 and published in 1770, describes a patient who had asthma for more than 10 years. The patient experienced acute attacks of asthma and had symptoms such as *shang qi* 上气, dyspnoea, rapid breathing, cough, phlegm, spontaneous sweating, cold limbs, and a deep and thin pulse. The patient was diagnosed with *qi* deficiency and Spleen deficiency and was treated with *Liu jun zi tang* 六君子汤. In the same book, another citation describes a patient with chronic asthma from a young age. The asthma was triggered by cold weather and symptoms included dyspnoea, cough, and phlegm. Treatment consisted of *Qing shang bu xia wan* 清上补下丸 plus *bei mu* 贝母, *tian men dong* 天门冬, *gan cao* 甘草, *jie geng* 桔梗, *gua lou* 瓜蒌, *huang lian* 黄连, and *huang qin* 黄芩.

The book *Shen Ju Ren Yi An* 沈菊人医案, written by *Shen Ju Ren* 沈菊人 and published in 1875, describes a male patient with asthma for five years. The patient had an acute attack of wind-cold and stagnation in the Lungs. The patient also had a hesitant, deficient, and thin pulse. To expel the wind-cold and tonify the deficiency, he was given *ban xia* 半夏, *gan cao* 甘草, *gui zhi* 桂枝, *ma huang* 麻黄, *sang bai pi* 桑白皮, *zi su zi* 紫苏子, *xing ren* 杏仁, and *bai guo* 白果.

Chinese Herbal Medicine

Most citations mentioned the use of Chinese herbal medicine treatments (869 citations, 89.5%), and herbal medicine plus acupuncture was used in treatments described by three citations (0.3%). There was a wide diversity of Chinese herbal medicine with a total of 566 unique formulae. Among these, a total of 444 formulae were only cited once, 68 cited twice, 24 cited three times, and 30 formulae were cited four or more times. The most common formulae were *She gan ma huang tang* 射干麻黄汤, *Xiao qing long tang* 小青龙汤, and *Ding chuan tang* 定喘汤 (Table 3.3). These formulae are still used to treat respiratory conditions including asthma in modern clinical practice by tonifying *qi* and releasing the exterior.

Most Frequent Herbs in Classical Literature Citations

Herbs were diverse and 413 unique herbs were cited. The top five herbs were *ban xia* 半夏, *xing ren* 杏仁, *gan cao* 甘草, *ma huang* 麻黄, and *fu ling* 茯苓 (Table 3.4). Herbs often had *qi*-regulating and phlegm-transforming properties. These herbs cited in classic literature are still used in modern clinical practice for asthma and other respiratory conditions.

Chinese Herbal Medicine Citations Related to Asthma

Quotes with a description of asthma symptoms and detailed formula or acupuncture points have been translated. These examples highlight representative citations for asthma found in the classical literature.

In the book *Jin Gui Yao Lue* 金匮要略 (c. 219), a citation describes a patient with cough, dyspnoea, and a wheezing sound in his throat; *She gan ma huang tang* 射干麻黄汤 was prescribed. In another book, *Zhou Hou Bei Ji Fang* 肘后备急方 (c. 363), *Bai qian tang* 白前汤 (originally from the book *Shen Shi Fang* 深师方) was used to treat chronic cough, dyspnoea, wheezing, swelling and fullness, and

Table 3.3 Most Frequent Formulae in Classical Literature Citations

Formula Name	Herb Ingredients	No. of Citations
She gan ma huang tang 射干麻黄汤	She gan 射干, ma huang 麻黄, sheng jiang 生姜, zi wan 紫菀, kuan dong hua 款冬花, xi xin 细辛, wu wei zi 五味子, ban xia 半夏, da zao 大枣	51
Xiao qing long tang 小青龙汤	Gan jiang 干姜, gui zhi 桂枝, jie geng 桔梗, ma huang 麻黄, zi su zi 紫苏子, xi xin 细辛, xing ren 杏仁	25
Ding chuan tang 定喘汤	Gan cao 甘草, bai guo 白果, huang qi 黄芪, kuan dong hua 款冬花, ma huang 麻黄, sang bai pi 桑白皮, ban xia 半夏, zi su zi 紫苏子, xing ren 杏仁	22
Bai qian tang 白前汤	Bai qian 白前, ban xia 半夏, jing da ji 京大戟, zi wan 紫菀	22
Liu jun zi tang 六君子汤	Ren shen 人参, ban xia 半夏, bai zhu 白术, chen pi 陈皮, fu ling 茯苓, gan cao 甘草	10
Ting li da zao xie fei tang 葶苈大枣泻肺汤	Da zao 大枣, ting li zi 葶苈子	10
Yue pi jia ban xia tang 越脾加半夏汤	Ban xia 半夏, ma huang 麻黄, gan cao 甘草	8
Hou pu ma huang tang 厚朴麻黄汤	Ban xia 半夏, gan jiang 干姜, hou po 厚朴, ma huang 麻黄, shi gao 石膏, wu wei zi 五味子, xi xin 细辛, xiao mai 小麦, xing ren 杏仁	7
Qing jin dan 清金丹	Lai fu zi 莱菔子, sheng jiang 生姜, zao jia 皂角	6
Bai guo ding chuan tang 白果定喘汤	Bai guo 白果, ban xia 半夏, kuan dong hua 款冬花, ma huang 麻黄, huang qin 黄芩, zi su zi 紫苏子, xing ren 杏仁, chuan pu 川朴, gan cao 甘草, sang bai pi 桑白皮	6
Jia wei gan ju tang 加味甘桔汤	Bai qian 白前, bai bu 百部, bei mu 贝母, fu ling 茯苓, gan cao 甘草, jie geng 桔梗, ju hong 橘红, xuan fu hua 旋复花	6
Xiao chuan fang 哮喘方	Sang bai pi 桑白皮, dan dou chi 淡豆豉, bai fan 白矾	6

Note: Ma huang tang 麻黄汤 was used in 20 citations; however, the ingredients varied and therefore it was not counted in the formula list. The use of some herbs such as ma huang may be restricted in some countries; readers are advised to comply with relevant regulations.

Table 3.4　Most Frequent Herbs in Classical Literature Citations

Herb Name	Scientific name	No. of Citations
Ban xia 半夏	*Pinellia ternata* (Thunb.) Breit.	232
Xing ren 杏仁	*Prunus armeniaca* L.	214
Gan cao 甘草	*Glycyrrhiza spp.*	210
Ma huang 麻黄	*Ephedra spp.*	165
Fu ling 茯苓	*Poria cocos* (Schw.) Wolf	145
Sheng jiang 生姜	*Zingiber officinale* Rosc.	112
Zi su zi 紫苏子	*Perilla frutescens* (L.) Britt.	89
Kuan dong hua 款冬花	*Tussilago farfara* L.	88
Sang bai pi 桑白皮	*Morus alba* L.	81
Chen pi 陈皮	*Citrus reticulata* Blanco	78
Wu wei zi 五味子	*Schisandra chinensis* (Turcz.) Baill.	76
Zi wan 紫菀	*Aster tartaricus* L.f.	72
Gan jiang 干姜	*Zingiber officinale* Rosc.	65
Bei mu 贝母*	*Fritillaria spp.*	62
Xi xin 细辛	*Asarum sieboldii* Miq. Var. seoulense Nakai	62
Da zao 大枣	*Ziziphus jujuba* Mill.	56
Huang qin 黄芩	*Scutellaria baicalensis* Georgi	56
Jie geng 桔梗	*Platycodon grandiflorum* (Jacq.) A. DC.	55
Bai guo 白果	*Ginkgo biloba* L.	52
Ju hong 橘红	*Citrus reticulata* Blanco	49

*Includes *chuan bei mu* and *zhe bei mu*. In the classical literature, some citations mentioned *chuan bei mu* and others only mentioned *bei mu*; therefore they are merged together as '*bei mu*.'

Note: The use of some herbs such as ma huang may be restricted in some countries; readers are advised to comply with relevant regulations.

difficulty with falling asleep. *Bai qian tang* 白前汤 included the herbs *bai qian* 白前, *zi wan* 紫菀, *ban xia* 半夏, and *da ji* 大戟.

In *Jin Gui Yi* 金匮翼 (c. 1749), the formula *Xiao qing long tang* 小青龙汤 (originally from *Shang Han Lun* 伤寒论) was used for wheezing caused by phlegm retention in the Lung, cold, wheezing and suffocation, difficulty lying flat, and exogenous cold and internal fluid. *Xiao qing long tang* 小青龙汤 included *ma huang* 麻黄, *gui zhi* 桂枝, *shao yao* 芍药, *xi xin* 细辛, *gan cao* 甘草, *gan jiang* 干姜, *ban xia* 半夏, and *wu wei zi* 五味子.

Another example published in *Yi Deng Xu Yan* 医灯续焰 in 1652 describes *San zi yang qin tang* 三子养亲汤 (originally from *Han Shi Yi Tong* 韩氏医通 and made of *su zi* 苏子, *bai jie zi* 白芥子, and *lai fu zi* 莱菔子) for treating elderly people with excessive phlegm and *qi*, as well as wheezing caused by *qi* stagnation.

Acupuncture and Related Therapies

Acupuncture citations were most commonly found in books from the Qing Dynasty (1645–1911). The earliest citations were found in the Han Dynasty from the book, *Zhen Jiu Jia Yi Jing* 针灸甲乙经, written by *Huang Fu Mi* 皇甫谧 and published around 259. These early citations mentioned KI26 *Yuzhong* 彧中 and ST9 *Renying* 人迎 for asthma. Classical literature citations mentioned 55 different acupuncture points. Points on the Conception Vessel, Stomach, and Bladder meridians were most common, yet all meridians were mentioned at least once, except for the Gallbladder meridian. The most common points were CV22 *Tiantu* 天突, ST36 *Zusanli* 足三里, CV17 *Danzhong* 膻中, and KI27 *Shufu* 俞府 (Table 3.5).

Moxibustion was mentioned in 26 citations, needle acupuncture in 16 citations, ginger moxibustion in eight, needles and moxibustion in seven, acupressure in two, and point application therapy in one. Thirty-three citations did not mention the acupuncture method. Acupuncture points that were commonly mentioned in the 93 citations were CV22 *Tiantu* 天突, ST36 *Zusanli* 足三里, and CV17 *Danzhong* 膻中.

All citations mentioned wheezing and dyspnoea, and acupuncture points were similar irrespective of the symptoms described. Citations that mentioned cough frequently included EX-HN-10 *Juquan* 聚泉, and sputum was commonly treated with KI27 *Shufu* 俞府, ST40 *Fenglong* 丰隆, ST36 *Zusanli* 足三里, and CV17 *Danzhong* 膻中.

Acupuncture Citations Related to Asthma

In the book *Zhen Jiu Ju Ying* 针灸聚英 published in 1529, CV20 *Huagai* 华盖 was used to treat rapid respiration, cough, wheezing,

Table 3.5 Most Frequent Acupuncture Points in Classical Literature Citations

Acupuncture Point	No. of Citations
CV22 Tiantu 天突	35
ST36 Zusanli 足三里	21
CV17 Danzhong 膻中	20
KI27 Shufu 俞府	18
BL13 Feishu 肺俞	12
ST18 Rugen 乳根	12
CV15 Jiuwei 鸠尾	9
CV21 Xuanji 璇玑	8
EX-HN-10 Juquan 聚泉	7
SI17 Tianrong 天容	7
BL43 Gaohuang 膏肓	6
KI26 Yuzhong 彧中	6
CV6 Qihai 气海	5
ST40 Fenglong 丰隆	5
ST9 Renying 人迎	5
CV12 Zhongwan 中脘	4
CV23 Lianquan 廉泉	4

and expectoration. *Zhen Jiu Jia Yi Jing* 针灸甲乙经 (c. 282) described the treatment of cough, profuse spittle, dyspnoea, wheezing, and restlessness with KI26 *Yuzhong* 彧中.

Chinese Herbal Medicine and Acupuncture

Three citations used CHM combined with acupuncture. Two citations described point application therapy and one citation described the use of moxibustion at BL13 *Feishu* 肺俞 to treat phlegm-type asthma with *Xiao qing long tang* 小青龙汤. The citations described wheezing and dyspnoea and two were used for asthma triggered by cold air.

Other Chinese Medicine Therapies

Six citations mentioned other CM therapies. They were found in books from the Song and Jin Dynasties (961–1271), Ming Dynasty (1369–1644), and Qing Dynasty (1645–1911). *Qigong* 气功 was described in two citations and techniques included lifting the waist and shaking the elbows. To regulate Lung *qi*, the patients rubbed their waist up and down and focused on directing their Lung *qi* through thought. The citation states that rubbing the waist and back can regulate *qi* movement and descend *qi*. Regulating Lung *qi* by thought can eliminate *qi* stagnation. In another citation, the *qigong* 气功 technique included squatting, pressing one foot with the hands and forcibly stretching the other foot, clicking the teeth, exhaling and inhaling, and swallowing saliva at 1 to 5am every day.

In four citations, the other therapies described are unconventional by today's standards and included nose-plugging with *bai guo* 白果 and *ma huang* 麻黄, smoking herbs in the nose and mouth, bathing the feet with cold water, and wearing clothes soaked in ginger juice. These citations provided little detail about the techniques used or the symptoms treated.

Classical Literature in Perspective

Classical literature written over the last 2,500 years provides important information that continues to guide modern clinical practice. Classical books include treatments for asthma and form the foundation knowledge of CM. The term 'asthma' and typical symptoms including wheezing, dyspnoea, cough, and phlegm were found in the classical literature. Citations were distributed throughout dynastic China (c. 206) until the Republic of China (1949) was established. Most citations were found in books written and published during the Ming Dynasty (1369–1644) and Qing Dynasty (1645–1911). Herbal medicine and acupuncture treatments have been consistently used over centuries and the common formulae, herbs, and acupuncture points are broadly consistent with treatments used for asthma in current guidelines and clinical practice.

There are many formulae and herbs that have been mentioned, but some were mentioned more frequently. Formulae such as *She gan ma huang tang* 射干麻黄汤, *Xiao qing long tang* 小青龙汤, and *Ding chuan tang* 定喘汤 were commonly used. Herbs such as *ban xia* 半夏, *xing ren* 杏仁, *gan cao* 甘草, *ma huang* 麻黄, and *fu ling* 茯苓 were also common in the classic literature. The frequently mentioned formulae and herbs are still used in modern CM practice.

Acupuncture points varied in classical citations reflecting the many different point combinations and individualised prescriptions. Acupuncture treatments for asthma have not changed significantly over time. Classical treatments often included CV22 *Tiantu* 天突, ST36 *Zusanli* 足三里, and CV17 *Danzhong* 膻中. *Qigong* 气功 was also reported in the classical literature and it is still used in clinical practice. Other rare CM therapies, such as smoking herbs and nose-plugging with herbs, appeared to be used for asthma but these other therapies are no longer used in modern CM practice.

The current review of the classical literature found that asthma was a common ailment for people in ancient China. Over thousands of years, physicians from different regions documented the use of herbal medicine and acupuncture for asthma. These results validate the currently used treatments and reflect the importance of classical literature in informing and guiding the treatment of asthma in CM today.

References

1. Zhang ZJ. Han Dynasty. Jin Gui Yao Lue. 2010. Shan Xi Science and Technology Press. [In Chinese: 汉. 张仲景. 金匮要略.]
2. Ge H. Zhou Hou Bei Ji Fang. c.363. [In Chinese: 东晋. 葛洪. 肘后备急方]
3. Chao YF. Zhu Bing Yuan Hou Lun. c.610. [In Chinese: 隋. 巢元方. 诸病源候论]
4. Sun SM. Bei Ji Qian Jin Yao Fang. c.652. [In Chinese: 唐. 孙思邈. 备急千金要方]
5. Sun SM. Qian Jin Yi Fang. c.682. [In Chinese: 唐. 孙思邈. 千金翼方]
6. Wang T. Wai Tai Mi Yao. c.752. [In Chinese: 唐. 王焘. 外台秘要]

7. Wang ZZ. Zhen Jiu Zi Shen Jin. c.1220. [In Chinese: 南宋. 王执中. 针灸资生经]

8. Zhang G. Yi Shuo. c.1224. [In Chinese: 南宋. 张杲. 医说]

9. Zhu ZH. Dan Xi Xin Fa. c.1481. [In Chinese: 元代. 朱丹溪. 丹溪心法]

10. Zhu ZH. Dan Xi Zhi Fa Xin Yao. c.1543. [In Chinese: 元代. 朱丹溪. 丹溪治法心要]

11. Yu T. Yi Xue Zheng Zhuan. c.1515. [In Chinese: 明. 虞抟. 医学正传]

12. Wang KT. Zheng Zhi Zhun Sheng. c.602. [In Chinese: 明. 王肯堂. 证治准绳]

13. Zhu L. Pu Ji Fang. c.1406. [In Chinese: 明. 朱棣. 普济方]

14. Lin PQ. Lei Zheng Zhi Cai. c.1839. [In Chinese: 清. 林珮琴. 类证治裁]

15. Hu R, editor. Zhong Hua Yi Dian [Encyclopaedia of Traditional Chinese Medicine]. 4th ed. Chengsha: Hunan Electronic and Audio-Visual Publishing House; 2000.

16. May BH, Lu CJ, Xue CCL. Collections of traditional Chinese medical literature as resources for systematic searches. J Altern Complement Med. 2012; **18**(12): 1101–1107. JACM-2011–0587.R2.

17. May BH, Lu YB, Lu CJ, Zhang AL, Chang S., Xue CCL. Systematic assessment of the representativeness of published collections of the traditional literature on Chinese Medicine. J Altern Complement Med. 2013; **19**(5): 403–9.

4

Method of Evaluating Clinical Evidence

OVERVIEW

This chapter describes the methods used to identify and evaluate a range of Chinese medicine interventions for asthma in clinical studies. Studies identified through a comprehensive search of medical databases were assessed against eligibility criteria. A review of the methodological quality of the studies was conducted using standardised methods. Results from the studies that were included in this review were evaluated to provide an estimate of the effects of a range of Chinese medicine therapies.

Introduction

The use of Chinese medicine (CM) for asthma has been well documented in the contemporary literature. This monograph examines the efficacy and safety of CM interventions for asthma in clinical studies. Interventions have been categorised as follows:

- Chinese herbal medicine (Chapter 5);
- Acupuncture and related therapies (Chapter 7);
- Other CM therapies (e.g., *qigong* 气功 and *tai chi* 推拿) (Chapter 8);
- Combination CM therapies (Chapter 9).

References to clinical trials were obtained and assessed by an expert group. Randomised controlled trials (RCT), controlled clinical trials (CCTs), and non-controlled studies were evaluated in detail. CCTs were evaluated using the same approach as RCTs and are described separately. Evidence from non-controlled studies is more difficult to evaluate; therefore, the approach adopted in this assessment was to describe the characteristics of the study, details of the intervention, and any adverse events. However, effects of interventions were not assessed. References to included studies are indicated by a letter followed by a number. Studies of Chinese herbal medicine are indicated by an "H," e.g. H1; studies of acupuncture and related therapies are indicated by an "A," e.g. A1; studies of other Chinese medicine therapies are indicated by an "O," e.g. O1; and combinations of Chinese medicine therapies (see Table 4.1) are indicated by a "C," e.g. C1.

Search Strategy

Evidence was gathered by searching in English and Chinese language databases and the methods followed the Cochrane Handbook of Systematic Reviews.[1] English language databases included PubMed, Excerpta Medica Database (Embase), Cumulative Index of Nursing and Allied Health Literature (CINAHL), Cochrane Central Register of Controlled Trials (CENTRAL) which includes the Cochrane Library, and Allied and Complementary Medicine Database (AMED). Chinese language databases included China BioMedical Literature (CBM), China National Knowledge Infrastructure (CNKI), Chonqing VIP (CQVIP), and Wanfang. Databases were searched from the date of their inception until May 2014. No restrictions were applied. Search terms were mapped to controlled vocabulary (where applicable) in addition to being searched as keywords.

To conduct a comprehensive search of the literature, the three search blocks for each intervention were combined using the search operator "AND" (or a database-specific variant), resulting in nine searches in each of the nine databases:

1. Reviews of Chinese herbal medicine (CHM);
2. Controlled trials of CHM (randomised and non-randomised);
3. Non-controlled studies of CHM;
4. Reviews of acupuncture and related therapies;
5. Controlled trials of acupuncture and related therapies (randomised and non-randomised);
6. Non-controlled studies of acupuncture and related therapies;
7. Reviews of other CM therapies;

8.   Controlled trials of other CM therapies (randomised and non-randomised);
9.   Non-controlled studies of other CM therapies.

Studies of combination CM therapies were identified through the above searches. In addition to electronic database searches, reference lists of systematic reviews and other included studies were searched for additional publications that may be relevant. Clinical trial registries were searched to identify clinical trials which were ongoing or completed, and where required, trial investigators were contacted to obtain their data. The searched trial registries included the Australian New Zealand Clinical Trial Registry (ANZCTR), the Chinese Clinical Trial Registry (ChiCTR), the EU Clinical Trials Register (EU-CTR), and USA National Institutes of Health register (ClinicalTrials.gov).

If required, trial investigators were contacted to obtain further information. Trial investigators were contacted by email or telephone and were followed up after two weeks if no reply was received. Where no response was received after one month, any unknown information was marked as not available.

Inclusion Criteria

- Participants: Studies including participants with a diagnosis of asthma according to The Global Initiative for Asthma (GINA),[2] Prevention and Treatment of Asthma Guidelines published by the Chinese Medical Association,[3] Practical Internal Medicine Asthma Diagnostic Criteria,[4] Internal Medicine Asthma Diagnostic Criteria,[5] Guiding Principles of Clinical Research on New Drugs of Traditional Chinese Medicine for Asthma,[6] or other diagnostic guidelines such as the European Respiratory Society/American Thoracic Society (ATS),[7] and symptoms, signs, and results from lung function tests;
- Studies including participants aged 18 years or older;
- Interventions: CHM, acupuncture and related therapies, or other CM therapies (see Table 4.1);
- Comparators: Placebo, no treatment, or pharmacotherapies that are routinely prescribed for asthma;
- Outcomes: Studies must report at least one of the pre-specified outcome measures (Table 4.2).

Table 4.1   CM Interventions Included in Clinical Evidence Evaluation

Category	Intervention
CHM	Oral CHM, Inhaled CHM, Topical CHM
Acupuncture and related therapies	Acupuncture, electroacupuncture, moxibustion, acupressure, ear acupressure, transcutaneous electrical nerve stimulation (TENS), hot compress of herbs on acupuncture points, ultrasonic leading, laser acupuncture, scalp acupuncture
Other Chinese medicine therapies	Tuina (Chinese massage), cupping, qigong

Abbreviations: CHM, Chinese herbal medicine; CM, Chinese medicine; TENS, transcutaneous electrical nerve stimulation.

Table 4.2   Outcomes

Outcome Categories	Outcome Measures	Scoring
Lung function	1. Forced expiratory volume in one second (FEV_1) 2. Forced vital capacity (FVC) 3. Peak expiratory flow (PEF)	1. L or %; higher is better 2. L or %; higher is better 3. L/s; higher is better
Health-related quality of life	Asthma Quality of Life Questionnaire (AQLQ)	1-7 points for each question; higher is better
Asthma control	Asthma Control Test (ACT)	5-25 points; higher is better
Exacerbation	Frequency	Number; lower is better
Rescue medication	Inhaled bronchodilator (β2-adrenoceptor agonists) use	Puffs/day; lower is better
Effective rate	1. Chinese Medicine Clinical Research Guidelines (中药新药临床研究指导原则)[6] 2. Traditional Chinese Medicine Syndrome Diagnostic Efficacy Standards (中医病证诊断疗效标准)[8] 3. Bronchial Asthma Guide (支气管哮喘防治指南)[9]	Number of people with improved symptoms and signs; higher is better
Adverse events	Number and type of adverse events	

Exclusion Criteria

- Studies without appropriate diagnostic criteria;
- Studies including children with asthma;
- Studies that included cough variant asthma or trials of medication-induced asthma, such as aspirin-induced asthma;
- Control, if pharmacotherapy, was not routinely prescribed for asthma;
- Studies using different pharmacotherapy co-interventions in the intervention and control groups.

Outcomes

Outcomes included validated measures recommended in asthma research guidelines as well as measures of clinical effects and adverse events (Table 4.2). Lung function is the main measure of airflow limitation in asthma. The primary lung function (spirometric) measures for asthma included forced expiratory volume in one second (FEV_1) and forced vital capacity (FVC). Increases of more than 0.23 L or 10% indicate a clinically important improvement.[9,10] Peak expiratory flow (PEF) was also measured.

Asthma-related quality of life was measured with the Asthma Quality of Life Questionnaire (AQLQ).[11] This questionnaire measures patients' impairment on a scale of one to seven; one indicating severe impairment and seven indicating no impairment. To assess asthma control, the Asthma Control Test (ACT) was evaluated.[12] ACT includes five items relating to shortness of breath, night-time waking, activity, rescue bronchodilator use, and rating of asthma control. Reduction in the frequency of asthma exacerbations is an important measure in asthma studies, and fewer exacerbations indicate better asthma control and reduced morbidity and mortality. Data on the number of exacerbations was evaluated over the study periods. Rescue bronchodilator use was measured as part of other questionnaires including the ACT; however, it was also evaluated as a standalone outcome in the included studies.

Effective rate is not a validated measure of treatment effect in asthma clinical trials. However, it does describe the number of patients that achieved a positive result as assessed by a study doctor. The three most common criteria for assessing effective rate in CM clinical trials are the Traditional Chinese Medicine Syndrome Diagnostic Efficacy Standards 中医病证诊断疗效标准, the Chinese Medicine Clinical Research Guidelines 中药新药临床研究指导原则, and the Bronchial Asthma Guide 支气管哮喘防治指南.[6,8,9] Patients that achieve a result are categorised into one of four groups:

1. Clinical control: Symptoms of asthma are either fully relieved or there is no longer a need to take asthma medications even if there are some occasional mild symptoms. FEV_1 or PEF increases by >35%, or FEV_1 (or PEF) is increased by ≥80% predicted after treatment. Variation rate of PEF between day and night is <20%;
2. Markedly effective: Symptoms of asthma are significantly relieved. FEV_1 or PEF increases by 25–35%, or FEV_1 (or PEF) is increased by 60–79% predicted after treatment. Variation rate of PEF between day and night >20% and the patient needs to use bronchodilators or glucocorticoids;
3. Effective: Symptoms of asthma are partially relieved. FEV_1 or PEF increases by 15–24% and the patient needs to use bronchodilators or glucocorticoids;
4. Ineffective: Symptoms and FEV_1 (or PEF) are not improved or become worse.

To analyse the effective rate outcome, all patients that had an improvement (i.e., clinical control, markedly effective, and effective) were grouped together. The pooled group was then compared to patients that did not experience any improvement (ineffective). Results were analysed using risk ratio (RR) with 95% confidence intervals (CI).

Risk of Bias Assessment

Risk of bias was assessed for RCTs using the Cochrane Collaboration's Risk of Bias Tool.[1] In clinical trials, bias can be categorised as selection bias, performance bias, detection bias, attrition bias, and reporting bias. Each domain is assessed to determine whether there is low, high, or unclear risk of bias. Low risk of bias indicates that bias is unlikely, whereas high risk indicates plausible bias that seriously weakens confidence in the results. Unclear bias indicates uncertainty or lack of information over the presence of potential bias and raises some doubt about the results. For the current review, the risk of bias assessment was conducted by two people and any disagreement was resolved by discussion and consultation with a third person.

Risk of bias is categorised using the following six domains:

- Sequence generation: The method used to generate the allocation sequence is given in sufficient detail to allow an assessment of whether it should produce comparable groups. Risk of bias is low when random number tables or computer random generators are used. High risk of bias includes studies that describe a non-random sequence generation, such as odd or even date of birth or date of admission.
- Allocation concealment: The method used to conceal the allocation sequence is given in enough detail to determine whether intervention allocations could have been foreseen before or during enrolment. Risk of bias is reduced when there is central randomisation or sealed envelopes are used, while bias risk is increased when open random sequences or date of birth, etc. are used.
- Blinding of participants and personnel: Measures used to describe if the study participants and personnel are blind to the intervention received. Information relating to whether the blinding was effective was additionally assessed. Studies that ensure blinding of participants and personnel have low risk of bias. If the participants and personnel in a study are not blinded, it has high risk of bias.
- Blinding of outcome assessors: Measures used to describe if the outcome assessors are blind to knowledge of which intervention a participant received. Additional assessment for the efficacy of the precautionary measure was performed as per the above point.
- Incomplete outcome data: Completeness of outcome data for each main outcome, including drop outs, exclusions from the analysis

with numbers missing in each group, and reasons for drop out or exclusions. Studies with low risk of bias would include all outcome data or, where data is missing, explain how this is unlikely to relate to the true outcome or is balanced between groups. Studies at high risk of bias would have unexplained missing data.

- Selective reporting: The study protocol is available and the pre-specified outcomes are included in the report. Studies with a published protocol and which include all pre-specified outcomes in their report would be at low risk of bias. Studies that do not include all pre-specified outcomes or the outcome data is reported incompletely have high risk of bias.

Statistical Analyses

Frequency of CM syndromes, CHM formulae, herbs, and acupuncture points reported in included studies are presented using descriptive statistics. CM syndromes reported in two or more studies are presented. The 10 most frequently reported CHM formulae and 20 most frequently reported herbs that are used in at least two studies are presented, although for CHM formulae this was not always possible. The top 20 acupuncture points used in two or more studies are presented, or as available. Where data was limited, reports of single CM syndromes or acupuncture points were provided as a guide for the reader.

Definitions of statistical tests and results are described in the glossary. Dichotomous data are reported as a risk ratio (RR) with 95% confidence intervals (CI), and continuous data are reported as mean difference (MD) with 95% CI. For all analyses, estimates of heterogeneity were reported with RR or MD and 95% CI. Formal tests for heterogeneity were conducted using the I^2 statistic. An I^2 score greater than 50% was taken to indicate substantial heterogeneity.[1] Sensitivity analyses were undertaken to explore potential sources of heterogeneity, based on low risk of bias for the risk of bias domain sequence generation. Where possible and appropriate, planned subgroup analyses included duration of treatment and CM interventions. Available case analysis with a random effects model was used in all analyses. The random effects model was used to take into account the clinical heterogeneity likely to be encountered within and between included studies, and the variation in treatment effects between included studies.

Assessment Using GRADE

The Grading of Recommendations Assessment, Development, and Evaluation (GRADE) approach was used.[10] The GRADE approach summarises and rates the quality of evidence in systematic reviews using a structured process for presenting evidence summaries. The results are summarised in tabular form which provides an important overview for asthma outcomes.

A panel of experts was established to evaluate the quality of evidence. The panel included the systematic review team, CM practitioners, integrative medicine experts, research methodologists, and conventional medicine physicians. The experts were asked to rate the clinical importance of key interventions from CHM, acupuncture therapies, and other CM therapies, as well as comparators and outcomes. Results were collated and a consensus on the content for the summary of findings tables was achieved based on the rating scores and subsequent discussion.

The quality of evidence for each outcome was rated according to five factors outlined in the GRADE approach. The quality of evidence may be rated down based on:

- Limitations in study design (risk of bias);
- Inconsistency of results (unexplained heterogeneity);
- Indirectness of evidence (interventions, populations, and outcomes important to the patients with the condition);
- Imprecision (uncertainty about the results);
- Publication bias (selective publication of studies).

These five factors are additive and a reduction in more than one factor will reduce the quality of the evidence for that outcome. The GRADE approach also includes three domains that can be rated up, including large magnitude of an effect, dose-response gradient, and effect of plausible residual confounding. However, these three domains relate to observational studies including cohort, case-control, before-after, time series studies, etc. GRADE summaries in this monograph only included RCTs and thus these three domains for rating up were not assessed.

Treatment recommendations can also be assessed using the GRADE approach, but due to the diverse nature of CM practice, treatment recommendations were not included with the summary of findings. Therefore, the reader is able to interpret the evidence with reference to the local practice environment. It should also be noted that the GRADE approach requires judgments about the quality of evidence and some subjective assessment. However, the experience of the panel members suggests that the judgments are reliable and thus serve as transparent representations of the quality of evidence.

The GRADE levels of evidence are grouped into four categories:

(1) High quality evidence: Further research is very unlikely to change our confidence in the estimate of effect.
(2) Moderate quality evidence: Further research is likely to have an important impact on our confidence in the estimate of effect and may change the estimate.
(3) Low quality evidence: Further research is very likely to have an important impact on our confidence in the estimate of effect and is likely to change the estimate.
(4) Very low quality evidence: Any estimate of reported effects is very uncertain.

References

1. Higgins JPT, Green S, editors: Cochrane Handbook for Systematic Reviews of Interventions Version 5.1.0 [updated March 2011]. The Cochrane Collaboration, 2011.
2. Global Strategy for Asthma Management and Prevention. (2015). Global Initiative for Asthma (GINA). Available from: http://www. ginasthma.org/.

3. 中华医学会呼吸病学分会哮喘学组. 支气管哮喘防治指南. 中华医学会呼吸病学分会哮喘学组. 支气管哮喘防治指南. Multiple editions available.

4. Chen HZ. Practical Internal Medicine. People's Medical Publishing House. [In Chinese: 陈灏珠. 实用内科学. 人民卫生出版社.] Multiple editions available.

5. 全国高等学校教材. 内科学. 人民卫生出版. 社 Multiple editions available.

6. Zhen XY. (2002) Guiding Principle of Clinical Research on New Drugs of Traditional Chinese Medicine. Chinese medical science and technology press. [In Chinese: 郑筱萸. 中药新药临床研究指导原则. 中国医药科技出版社].

7. Chung KF, Wenzel SE, Brozek JL, Bush A, Castro M, Sterk PJ, *et al*. (2014) International ERS/ATS guidelines on definition, evaluation and treatment of severe asthma. Eur Respir J. **43**(2):343–73.

8. 中华人民共和国中医药行业标准. 国家中医药管理局发布. 中医病证诊断疗效标准. 1994.

9. Prevention and treatment of asthma guideline. (1997) Chin J Tuberc Respir Dis, 20(5):261–267. [In Chinese: 支气管哮喘防治指南. 中华结核和呼吸杂志, 1997;**20**(5):261–267].

10. Schünemann H, Brożek J, Guyatt G, Oxman A, editors. (2013) GRADE handbook for grading quality of evidence and strength of recommendations. Updated October 2013. The GRADE Working Group, 2013. Available from www.guidelinedevelopment.org/handbook.

11. Juniper EF, Guyatt GH, Willan A, Griffith LE. (1994) Determining a minimal important change in a disease-specific quality of life questionnaire. J Clin Epidemiol **47**(1):81–87.

12. Schatz M, Kosinski M, Yarlas AS, Hanlon J, Watson ME, Jhingran P. (2009) The minimally important difference of the Asthma Control Test. J Allergy Clin Immunol **124**:719–23.

5

Clinical Evidence for Chinese Herbal Medicine

OVERVIEW

Chinese herbal medicine for asthma has been widely studied in clinical trials. This chapter provides an up-to-date synopsis and analysis of the clinical trial literature. Nine scientific databases identified over 20,000 citations. Rigorous criteria were applied and irrelevant studies were excluded. A total of 333 clinical studies investigated CHM for chronic asthma and acute exacerbations of asthma. Evidence is promising and Chinese herbal medicine, either alone or when combined with routine asthma pharmacotherapies, improved lung function, asthma control, health-related quality of life, exacerbation frequency, use of rescue medication, and effective rate.

Introduction

Chinese herbal medicine (CHM) is used for asthma and has been researched in clinical trials. A systematic review and a series of meta-analyses were performed to determine the efficacy and safety of CHM for adult asthma. Many different formulae and herb combinations were evaluated for the treatment of asthma, and the formulae and herb combinations that are most commonly evaluated in clinical trials are presented in this chapter. Included studies are indicated by an "H" followed by a number, e.g. (H1). The reference list for included studies can be found at the end of this chapter.

Previous Systematic Reviews

CHM has been evaluated in several reviews and discussion articles and yet only two systematic reviews have been published. In 2000, Huntley *et al.* showed mixed results of CHM for asthma.[1] Two studies using *bai guo* 白果 and invigorating Kidney herbs improved lung function but other CHM such as *chuan xiong* 川芎, tonifying herbs, and *Wan yang tong luo he ji* 温阳通络合剂 did not produce an effect that was greater than the control group. The authors could not draw any firm conclusions because of variability in the CHM interventions and poorly designed studies, including no blinding or lack of randomisation. In 2008, Arnold *et al.* published a review in Cochrane.[2] From the 29 studies included, two reported improvements in lung function and one reported improvements in health-related quality of life. Unfortunately, the authors could not show whether the herbal treatments improved asthma symptoms due to differences in study design, methodological shortfalls, and limited use of validated outcomes. In 2014, Hong *et al.* published an article on the effects and mechanisms of CHM for asthma.[3] They concluded that CHMs have broad effects on asthma mechanisms, noting that CHM may benefit patients with corticosteroid resistant asthma and further research may eventually prove that CHM can be effectively used as monotherapy or as integrative therapy for asthma.

Characteristics of Chinese Herbal Medicine Clinical Studies

A search of English and Chinese databases identified 28,153 citations. After excluding duplicates, 18,684 were screened and 1,429 underwent full-text review (Figure 5.1). After all exclusions, CHM for asthma was examined in 333 clinical studies (H1–H333). A total of 246 were randomised controlled trials (RCTs), 18 were controlled clinical trials, and 69 were non-controlled studies (Figure 5.1). Majority of these studies were conducted in China, but some studies were also conducted in Japan, USA, and the UK. Evidence from RCTs are pooled in meta-analyses to provide evidence for CHM treatments,

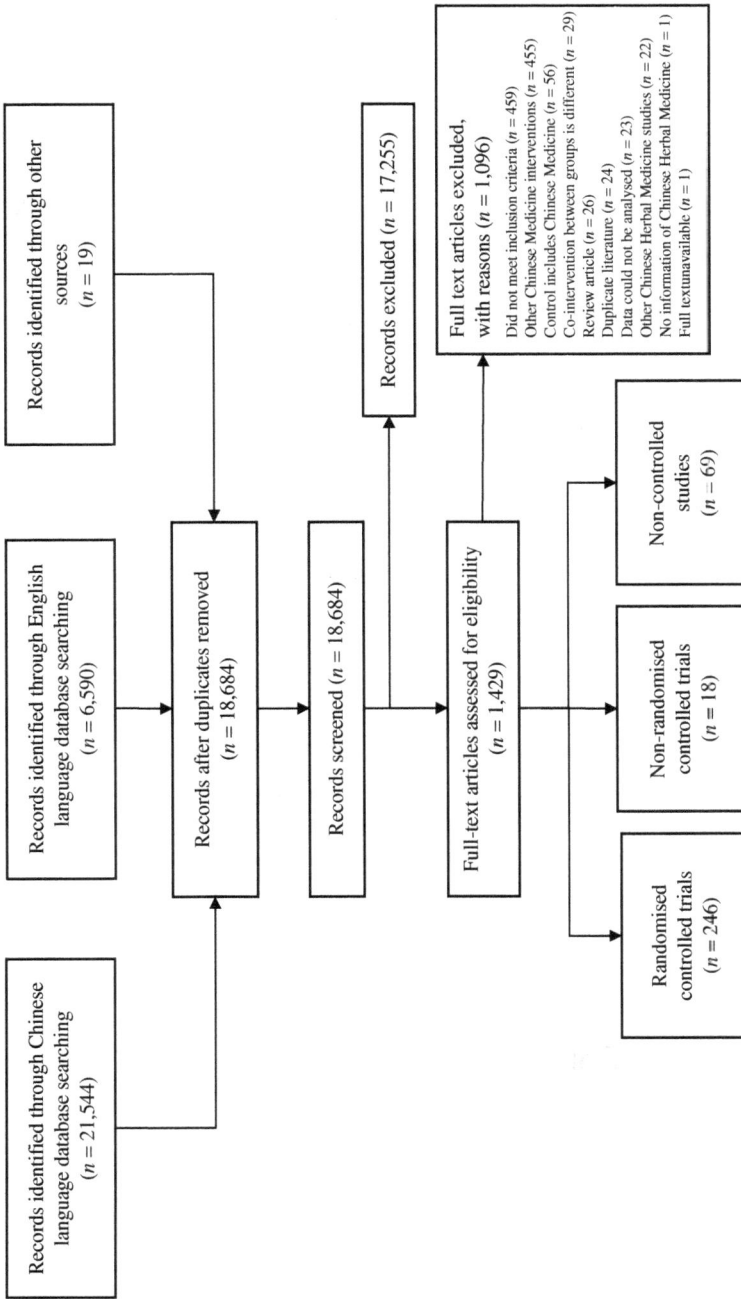

Figure 5.1. Flow chart of study selection process: Chinese herbal medicine.

Records identified through Chinese language database searching
($n = 21,544$)

Records identified through English language database searching
($n = 6,590$)

Records identified through other sources
($n = 19$)

Records after duplicates removed
($n = 18,684$)

Records screened ($n = 18,684$)

Records excluded ($n = 17,255$)

Full-text articles assessed for eligibility
($n = 1,429$)

Full text articles excluded, with reasons ($n = 1,096$)

Did not meet inclusion criteria ($n = 459$)
Other Chinese Medicine interventions ($n = 455$)
Control includes Chinese Medicine ($n = 56$)
Co-intervention between groups is different ($n = 29$)
Review article ($n = 26$)
Duplicate literature ($n = 24$)
Data could not be analysed ($n = 23$)
Other Chinese Herbal Medicine studies ($n = 22$)
No information of Chinese Herbal Medicine ($n = 1$)
Full textunavailable ($n = 1$)

Randomised controlled trials
($n = 246$)

Non-randomised controlled trials
($n = 18$)

Non-controlled studies
($n = 69$)

with the same approach used for controlled clinical trials. Other study types such as case series are qualitatively summarised but their results are not included in the evidence analysis.

A large number of participants (n = 27,315) were evaluated in these studies. Asthma duration ranged from six months to 55 years and treatment duration ranged from seven days to three years. Most commonly, CHM was administered as decoction, although capsules, tablets, and granules were also regularly used. CHM was less commonly prepared as a nebulised liquid and inhaled or topically applied.

CHM treatments included over 193 different formulae and 262 different herbs. The most common formulae were *Xiao qing long tang* 小青龙汤, *Ding chuan tang* 定喘汤, *She gan ma huang tang* 射干麻黄汤, and *Ma xing shi gan tang* 麻杏石甘汤. The most common herbs were *ma huang* 麻黄, *gan cao* 甘草, *xing ren* 杏仁, and *ban xia* 半夏 (Table 5.1 and 5.2). CHM was administered orally, inhaled, or applied topically as an external ointment. Included studies compared CHM to placebos, pharmacotherapy, and no treatment, and also compared CHM combined with pharmacotherapy to pharmacotherapy alone (integrative medicine). Pharmacotherapies mostly included bronchodilators, corticosteroids, and their combinations. Studies that defined the CM syndromes included phlegm-cold or phlegm-heat (41 studies), Kidney deficiency (10 studies), phlegm obstructing the Lung (nine studies), Lung, Spleen, and Kidney deficiency (six studies), wind-phlegm obstructing the Lung (four studies), and Lung and Kidney deficiency and wind-cold or heat attacking the Lung (four studies).

Randomised Controlled Trials of Chinese Herbal Medicine

CHM for adult asthma was evaluated in 246 RCTs conducted on 21,394 participants (H1–H246). Studies were separated into two categories, chronic asthma (124 studies, 11,082 participants) and acute exacerbations of asthma (122 studies, 10,312 participants).

Table 5.1   Frequently Reported Formulae in all CHM Clinical Studies

Formulae Name	No. of Studies	Ingredients
Xiao qing long tang 小青龙汤	18	Ma huang 麻黄, gui zhi 桂枝, shao yao 芍药, gan cao 甘草, gan jiang 干姜, xi xin 细辛, ban xia 半夏, wu wei zi 五味子
Ding chuan tang 定喘汤	11	Bai guo 白果, ma huang 麻黄, sang bai pi 桑白皮, kuan dong hua 款冬花, ban xia 半夏, xing ren 杏仁, zi su zi 紫苏子, huang qin 黄芩, gan cao 甘草
She gan ma huang tang 射干麻黄汤	10	She gan 射干, ma huang 麻黄, xi xin 细辛, zi wan 紫菀, kuan dong hua 款冬花, ban xia 半夏, wu wei zi 五味子, sheng jiang 生姜, da zao 大枣
Ma xing shi gan tang 麻杏石甘汤	7	Ma huang 麻黄, xing ren 杏仁, shi gao 石膏, gan cao 甘草
Bu zhong yi qi tang 补中益气汤	5	Ren shen 人参, huang qi 黄芪, bai zhu 白术, gan cao甘草, dang gui 当归, chen pi 陈皮, sheng ma 升麻, chai hu 柴胡
San zi yang qin tang 三子养亲汤	4	Zi su zi 紫苏子, bai jie zi 白芥子, lai fu zi 莱服子

Ingredients are referenced to the *Zhong Yi Fang Ji Da Ci Dian* 中医方剂大辞典 where available, or to the included study if not available.

Note: The use of some herbs such as ma huang may be restricted in some countries; readers are advised to comply with relevant regulations.

Formulae were diverse and 130 different formulae were researched. The most common were *Xiao qing long tang* 小青龙汤, *Ding chuan tang* 定喘汤, and *She gan ma huang tang* 射干麻黄汤 (Table 5.3). Herbs were also diverse and 210 different herbs were included in the formulae. The most common were *ma huang* 麻黄, *gan cao* 甘草, *xing ren* 杏仁, and *ban xia* 半夏 (Table 5.4). Formulae were given orally in 239 studies (i.e., decoction, pills, capsules, and granules), inhaled in five studies, and applied topically in two studies.

Table 5.2   Frequently Reported Herbs in all Clinical Studies

Herb Name	Scientific Name	No. of Studies
Ma huang 麻黄	*Ephedra spp.*	183
Gan cao 甘草	*Glycyrrhiza spp.*	161
Xing ren 杏仁	*Prunus armeniaca* L.	126
Ban xia 半夏	*Pinellia ternata* (Thunb.) Breit.	117
Di long 地龙	*Pheretima spp.*	94
Wu wei zi 五味子	*Schisandra chinensis* (Turcz.) Baill.	87
Huang qin 黄芩	*Scutellaria baicalensis* Georgi	80
Zi su zi 紫苏子	*Perilla frutescens* (L.) Britt.	68
Xi xin 细辛	*Asarum spp.*	63
Huang qi 黄芪	*Astragalus membranaceus* (Fisch.) Bge.	59
Chen pi 陈皮	*Citrus reticulata* Blanco	57
Fu ling 茯苓	*Poria cocos* (Schw.) Wolf	53
Kuan dong hua 款冬花	*Tussilago farfara* L.	49
Bai shao 白芍	*Paeonia lactiflora* Pall.	46
Sang bai pi 桑白皮	*Morus alba* L.	43
Chan tui 蝉蜕	*Cryptotympana pustulata* Fabricius	43
Ting li zi 葶苈子	*Lepidium apetalum* Willd., *Descurainia sophia* (L.) Webb. ex Prantl.	43
Zi wan 紫菀	*Aster tataricus* L. f.	40
Dan shen 丹参	*Salvia miltiorrhiza* Bge.	39
Bai jie zi 白芥子	*Brassica juncea* (L.) Czern. & Coss.or *Sinapis alba* L.	37
Bai zhu 白术	*Atractylodes macrocephala* Koidz.	37
She gan 射干	*Belamcanda chinensis* (L.)DC.	37

Note: The use of some herbs such as ma huang may be restrieted in some countries; readers are advised to comply with relevant regulations.

Duration of asthma ranged from six months to 48 years and participants' average age was 45 years. There were 10,732 male and 8,863 female participants (the sex of 1,799 participants was not stated). CM syndromes were described in 90 studies. Common

Table 5.3 Frequently Reported Formulae in RCTs

Asthma Stage	Formulae Name	No. of Studies	Ingredients
Acute	Xiao qing long tang 小青龙汤	12	Ma huang 麻黄, gui zhi 桂枝, shao yao 芍药, gan cao 甘草, gan jiang 干姜, xi x n 细辛, ban xia 半夏, wu wei zi 五味子
	She gan ma huang tang 射干麻黄汤	6	She gan 射干, ma huang 麻黄, xi xin 细辛, zi wan 紫菀, kuan dong hua 款冬花, ban xia 半夏, wu wei zi 五味子, sheng jiang 生姜, da zao 大枣
	Ding chuan tang 定喘汤	3	Bai guo 白果, ma huang 麻黄, sang bai pi 桑白皮, kuan dong hua 款冬花, ban xia 半夏, xing ren 杏仁, zi su zi 紫苏子, huang qin 黄芩, gan cao 甘草
	Ma xing shi gan tang 麻杏石甘汤	3	Ma huang 麻黄, xing ren 杏仁, shi gao 石膏, gan cao 甘草
Chronic	Bu zhong yi qi tang 补中益气汤	4	Ren shen 人参, huang qi 黄芪, bai zhu 白术, gan cao 甘草, dang gui 当归, chen pi 陈皮, sheng ma 升麻, chai hu 柴胡
	Ding chuan tang 定喘汤	3	Bai guo 白果, ma huang 麻黄, sang bai pi 桑白皮, kuan dong hua 款冬花, ban xia 半夏, xing ren 杏仁, zi su zi 紫苏子, huang qin 黄芩, gan cao 甘草
	Jin gui shen qi wan 金匮肾气丸	3	Gui zhi 桂枝, fu zi 附子, gan di huang 干地黄, shan zhu yu 山茱萸, shan yao 芍药, fu ling 茯苓, mu dan pi 牡丹皮, ze xie 泽泻
	Ma xing shi gan tang 麻杏石甘汤	3	Ma huang 麻黄, xing ren 杏仁, shi gao 石膏, gan cao 甘草

Ingredients are referenced to the *Zhong Yi Fang Ji Da Ci Dian* 中医方剂大辞典 where available, or to the included study if not available.

Note: The use of some herbs such as ma huang may be restrieted in some countries; readers are advised to comply with relevant regulations.

syndromes for acute asthma included phlegm-cold, phlegm-heat, phlegm-wind, and phlegm obstructing the Lung. For chronic asthma, syndromes were phlegm-cold, phlegm-heat, phlegm-wind, Kidney deficiency, phlegm obstructing the Lung, Lung,

Table 5.4 Frequently Reported Herbs in RCTs

Herb Name	Scientific Name	No. of Studies	Asthma Stage (No. of Studies)
Ma huang 麻黄	*Ephedra spp.*	131	C(47); A(84)
Gan cao 甘草	*Glycyrrhiza spp.*	121	C(56); A(65)
Xing ren 杏仁	*Prunus armeniaca* L.	91	C(35); A(56)
Ban xia 半夏	*Pinellia ternate* (Thunb.) Breit.	83	C(23); A(60)
Di long 地龙	*Pheretima spp.*	71	C(32); A(39)
Zi su zi 紫苏子	*Perilla frutescens* (L.) Britt.	67	C(24); A(43)
Huang qin 黄芩	*Scutellaria baicalensis* Georgi	65	C(23); A(42)
Wu wei zi 五味子	*Schisandra chinensis* (Turcz.) Baill.	65	C(27); A(38)
Xi xin 细辛	*Asarum spp.*	48	C(13); A(35)
Huang qi 黄芪	*Astragalus membranaceus* (Fisch.) Bge.	43	C(31); A(12)
Fu ling 茯苓	*Poria cocos* (Schw.) Wolf	39	C(21); A(18)
Chen pi 陈皮	*Citrus reticulata* Blanco	37	C(16); A(21)
Ting li zi 葶苈子	*Lepidium apetalum* Willd., *Descurainia sophia* (L.) Webb. ex Prantl.	35	C(12); A(23)
Chan tui 蝉蜕	*Cryptotympana pustulata* Fabricius	32	C(11); A(21)
Kuan dong hua 款冬花	*Tussilago farfara* L.	32	C(11); A(21)
Bai shao 白芍	*Paeonia lactiflora* Pall.	31	C(7); A(24)
Sang bai pi 桑白皮	*Morus alba* L.	31	C(11); A(20)
She gan 射干	*Belamcanda chinensis* (L.) DC.	29	C(7); A(22)
Dan shen 丹参	*Salvia miltiorrhiza* Bge.	28	C(11); A(17)
Zi wan 紫菀	*Aster tataricus* L. f.	28	C(9); A(19)

Abbreviations: A, acute exacerbations of asthma; C, chronic asthma.

Note: The use of some herbs such as ma huang may be restrieted in some contries; readers are advised to comply with relevant regulations.

Spleen, and Kidney deficiency, Lung *qi* deficiency, and Spleen *qi* deficiency.

Comparators include pharmacotherapy (231 studies), placebo (14 studies), and no treatment (one study). CHM plus pharmacotherapy (integrative medicine) compared to pharmacotherapy alone was evaluated in 167 studies.

Risk of Bias

All studies were randomised and 35 reported an appropriate method for sequence generation and only two reported allocation concealment (H205–H241). In five studies, sequence generation was at high risk of bias because they used quasi-randomised methods such as allocation by sequential numbering or allocation based on outpatient number (H2, H53, H83, H223, H244). There was adequate blinding of participants in 13 studies (5.3%), adequate blinding of personnel in eight studies, and blinding of outcome assessors in 17 studies which reduced the risk of bias; the other studies that did not adequately carry out blinding procedures faced higher bias risks. Outcome data was mostly at low risk of bias; 21 studies did not report details about loss to follow-up and were judged at unclear risk of bias, and one study was at high risk of bias because there was a large loss to follow-up without explanations. Most studies were at unclear risk of bias for selective outcome reporting because protocols were not available. Twenty-three were at high risk of bias because not all pre-specified outcomes were reported or outcomes were reported incompletely. Overall, the methodological quality was low (Table 5.5).

Table 5.5   Risk of Bias of RCTs: CHM

Risk of Bias Domain	Low Risk n (%)	Unclear Risk n (%)	High Risk n (%)
Sequence generation	35 (14.2%)	206 (83.7%)	5 (2.0%)
Allocation concealment	2 (0.8%)	244 (99.2%)	0
Blinding of participants	13 (5.3%)	1 (0.4%)	232 (94.3%)
Blinding of personnel	8 (3.3%)	2 (0.8%)	236 (95.9%)
Blinding of outcome assessors	17 (6.9%)	10 (4.1%)	219 (89.0%)
Incomplete outcome data	224 (91.1%)	21 (8.5%)	1 (0.4%)
Selective outcome reporting	0	223 (90.6%)	23 (9.3%)

Outcomes

The most common outcome was effective rate[4–6] reported in 212 studies (86.2%). Twenty-eight different definitions of effective rate were used and the most common definition was from the Bronchial Asthma Guide[6] used in 60 studies. Lung function forced expiratory volume in one second (FEV_1) was reported in 122 studies, forced vital capacity (FVC) in 33 studies, and PEF in 80 studies. The Asthma Control Test (ACT)[7] was reported in 16 studies and other outcomes were seldom used. Exacerbation of asthma in was documented in eight studies, use of rescue medication in eight studies, and Asthma Quality of Life Questionnaire (AQLQ)[8] in four studies. Adverse events were reported in 43 studies. Studies assessing acute asthma used effective rate as an outcome (115 studies, 94.3%) more often than chronic asthma studies (97 studies, 78.2%). Chronic asthma studies commonly evaluated lung function FEV_1 (64 studies, 51.6%) compared to acute asthma studies (58 studies, 47.5%). Acute studies did not use quality of life outcomes and only one evaluated use of rescue medication.

Chronic Asthma

Lung Function

CHM alone or combined with pharmacotherapy compared to pharmacotherapy alone improved lung function in people with chronic asthma. CHM alone improved lung function FEV_1% by 7.19% ([3.64, 10.74], I^2 = 80%); FEV_1L by 0.23L ([0.09, 0.37], I^2 = 58%); and FVC by 0.14L ([0.03, 0.26], I^2 = 0%) (Table 5.6). When CHM was combined with pharmacotherapy, FEV_1% improved by 7.14% ([5.24, 9.03], I^2 = 72%); FEV_1L by 0.38 L ([0.28, 0.49], I^2 = 71%); and FVC by 0.41L ([0.20, 0.62], I^2 = 77%) and 5.16% ([2.16, 8.17], I^2 = 0%), (Table 5.6). While the results are positive, there was heterogeneity in the data, and heterogeneity still remained high after sub-group analyses.

Compared to pharmacotherapy, peak expiratory flow was not improved by CHM (MD 0.23 [–0.10, 0.55], I^2 = 74%), but was

Table 5.6   Oral CHM — Lung Function (Chronic Asthma)

Comparator	Outcome	No. of Studies	No. of Participants	Effect Size MD [95% CI]	I² %	Included Studies
Pharmacotherapy	FEV₁%	11	900	7.19 [3.64, 10.74]*	80	H1, H5, H9, H31, H46, H48, H50, H52, H57, H61, H73
Pharmacotherapy	FEV₁ L	12	879	0.23 [0.09, 0.37]*	58	H1, H4, H5, H8, H19, H21, H28, H30, H34, H36, H66, H73
Pharmacotherapy	FVC L	8	585	0.14 [0.03, 0.26]*	0	H1, H5, H8, H19, H28, H30, H32, H66
Pharmacotherapy	PEF L/s	9	672	0.23 [−0.10, 0.55]	74	H1, H4, H5, H8, H21, H28, H35, H57, H65
Integrative medicine	FEV₁%	21	2283	7.14 [5.24, 9.03]*	72	H81, H103, H108, H111, H124, H127, H134, H147, H151, H154, H159, H168, H174, H182, H185, H190, H191, H193, H205, H222, H243
Integrative medicine	FEV₁ L	16	1121	0.38 [0.28, 0.49]*	71	H97, H99, H148, H149, H152, H154, H157, H163, H167, H180, H182, H208, H211, H222, H244, H245
Integrative medicine	FVC L	8	601	0.41 [0.20, 0.62]*	77	H97, H148, H149, H154, H157, H163, H222, H244
Integrative medicine	FVC%	4	377	5.16 [2.16, 8.17]*	0	H124, H127, H190, H191
Integrative medicine	PEF L/s	14	1562	0.83 [0.47, 1.19]*	94	H97, H108, H111, H124, H148, H154, H157, H163, H167, H180, H203, H211, H244, H245
Integrative medicine	PEF %	9	717	6.73 [2.47, 10.99]*	81	H127, H134, H151, H152, H160, H174, H190, H191, H244

*Statistically significant

Abbreviations: FEV₁, Forced Expiratory Volume in One Second; FVC, Forced Vital Capacity; PEF; Peak Expiratory Flow.

improved when CHM was combined with pharmacotherapy. PEF improved by 0.83 L/s ([0.47, 1.19], I^2 = 94%) and PEF% by 6.73% ([2.47, 10.99], I^2 = 81%) (Table 5.6). Results did not show any improvement when CHM was compared with placebos in two studies (FEV$_1$% mean difference (MD 2.87% [−1.96, 7.70], I^2 = 0%) (H40, H65). In meta-analyses that show positive results, the most common herbs were *gan cao* 甘草, *ma huang* 麻黄, *di long* 地龙, *xing ren* 杏仁, *huang qi* 黄芪, and *wu wei zi* 五味子.

Health-related Quality of Life

Few studies assessed health-related quality of life. One study assessed the participants' quality of life with the AQLQ after 12 weeks of CHM plus inhaled steroids and found that AQLQ scores showed no improvement (MD 2.22 points, [−2.30, 6.74] (H205).

Asthma Control

Asthma control measured with the ACT was evaluated in seven studies. In a single study comparing *Bu fei ke li* 补肺颗粒 to a placebo, the ACT improved by 1.55 points [0.52, 2.58] (H40). Five studies were pooled in a meta-analysis comparing CHM plus β2-adrenoceptor agonists (beta2-agonists) and steroids with beta2-agonists and steroids alone. CHM improved asthma control by 2.47 points (1.64, 3.29], I^2 = 55%) (H99, H103, H146, H157, H238). One study applied *Wen shen xiao chuan gao fang* 温肾消喘膏方 externally and the ACT in the intervention group improved compared to the control group (MD 0.91 points [0.10, 1.72] (H138).

Exacerbation Frequency

Exacerbation frequency was reported in four studies (H39, H100, H138, H238). Results could not be pooled because the duration of follow-up and the definition of frequency was different amongst studies. In a single study evaluating CHM plus pharmacotherapy compared with pharmacotherapy alone, exacerbation frequency reduced by −1.20 exacerbations per year [−1.82, −0.58] (H238). In another study comparing *Yi qi gu fei shu feng tang* 益气固肺疏风汤 to a placebo, frequency reduced by 1.90 exacerbations per year [−3.46, −0.34] (H39); similarly *Liu jun zi wan* 六君子丸 reduced frequency by −2.20 exacerbations over nine months [−2.70, −1.70] (H100). When an external CHM ointment plus pharmacotherapy was compared with pharmacotherapy alone for four months, the number of exacerbations reduced by 1.36 [−1.99, −0.73] (H138).

Use of Rescue Medication

Use of rescue medication was evaluated in two studies (H167, H205). Both studies evaluated the amount of salbutamol used. Results of single studies showed that *Zhi bai di huang wan* 知柏地黄丸 plus *Jin shui liu jun jian* 金水六君煎 plus budesonide compared with budesonide alone reduced the use of salbutamol (MD −1.72 puffs [−2.30, −1.14]) (H167). *Qing fei ping chuan bu shen ke li* 清肺平喘补肾颗粒 plus fluticasone/salmeterol compared with fluticasone/salmeterol alone also reduced salbutamol by 0.64 puffs [−0.79, −0.49] (H205).

Effective Rate

The ratings provided by investigators based on asthma symptoms served as a measure of the effective rate, or proportion of participants who achieved an improvement, and was evaluated in the majority of studies. The assessments of patient symptoms were performed by study doctors. Effective rate was defined by three guidelines, namely the Traditional Chinese Medicine (TCM) Syndrome Diagnostic Efficacy Standards, the Chinese Medicine Clinical Research Guidelines, and the Bronchial Asthma Guide. Compared with pharmacotherapy, CHM improved the effective rate according to the TCM Syndrome and Bronchial Asthma Guide criteria but not the Chinese Medicine Clinical Research Guideline. The largest effect and clinical improvement in the treatment group was 1.18 times that of the control group ([1.08, 1.30], $I^2 = 0\%$) (Table 5.7). The most frequent herbs

Table 5.7   Oral CHM — Effective Rate (Chronic Asthuma)

Comparator	Outcome — Effective Rate	No. of Studies	No. of Participants	Effect Size RR [95% CI]	I² %	Included Studies
Pharmacotherapy	Bronchial Asthma Guide	7	491	1.17 [1.01, 1.36]*	62	H1, H4, H5, H45, H60, H61, H71
Pharmacotherapy	CM Clinical Research Guidelines	9	675	1.05 [0.93, 1.19]	70	H6, H8, H11, H21, H29, H31, H32, H35, H52
Pharmacotherapy	TCM Syndrome Diagnostic Efficacy Standards	3	300	1.18 [1.08, 1.30]*	0	H3, H22, H27
Integrative medicine	Bronchial Asthma Guide	12	1112	1.20 [1.14, 1.26]*	0	H81, H92, H119, H127, H133, H151, H157, H161, H192, H193, H209, H211
Integrative medicine	CM Clinical Research Guidelines	7	491	1.19 [1.05, 1.35]*	81	H108, H111, H115, H124, H148, H149, H160

*Statistically significant
Abbreviations: CHM, Chinese Herbal Medicine; CM, Chinese Medicine; TCM, Traditional Chinese Medicine; RR, risk ratio.

in positive meta-analyses were *ma huang* 麻黄, *gan cao* 甘草, *jiang can* 僵蚕, and *di long* 地龙.

When CHM combined with pharmacotherapy was compared to pharmacotherapy alone, effective rate was improved based on the Bronchial Asthma Guide and the Chinese Medicine Clinical Research Guidelines. The chance of achieving a clinical improvement in the treatment group was 1.20 times that of the control group ([1.14, 1.26], $I^2 = 0\%$) with the Bronchial Asthma Guide. With the Chinese Medicine Clinical Research Guidelines, a similar finding was seen (RR 1.19 [1.05, 1.35], $I^2 = 81\%$) (Table 5.7).

Assessment Using GRADE: Chronic Asthma

Two GRADE summary of findings tables represent the main comparisons for chronic asthma. One compared CHM with placebo and the other compared CHM plus pharmacotherapy to pharmacotherapy alone.

Evidence for the effectiveness of CHM compared to a placebo was of moderate quality (Table 5.8). One study used *Bu fei ke li* 补肺颗粒 and the other used *ru xiang* 乳香, *jiang huang* 姜黄, and *gan cao* 甘草. The result was not statistically significant for $FEV_1\%$ but was significant for asthma control. Lung function PEF L/s, rescue bronchodilator use, exacerbation frequency, and quality of life were not measured.

Evidence for the effectiveness of CHM plus pharmacotherapy compared to pharmacotherapy alone ranged from very low to low quality (Table 5.9). The result was statistically significant for $FEV_1\%$, PEF L/s, asthma control, rescue bronchodilator use, and exacerbation frequency. Quality of life was not statistically different.

Randomised Controlled Trial Evidence from Individual Formula and Formula Commonly Used in Clinical Practice

Bu zhong yi qi tang 补中益气汤 plus pharmacotherapy versus pharmacotherapy alone improved the effective rate in two studies according to the Bronchial Asthma Guide (RR 1.21 [1.04, 1.38], $I^2 =$ 0%) (H127, H133). This result shows that *Bu zhong yi qi tang* 补中益气汤 improved asthma similarly, but the effect is not greater than that of all CHMs.

Assessment Using GRADE

The main formula for asthma based on number of RCTs and expert opinion is presented in a GRADE summary of findings table. Evidence for the effectiveness of *Bu zhong yi qi tang* 补中益气汤 plus pharmacotherapy compared to pharmacotherapy was of low quality (Table 5.10). The result was not statistically significant for $FEV_1\%$. Other outcomes were not reported.

Table 5.8   GRADE: CHM vs. Placebo for Chronic Asthma

Outcomes and Follow-up	No. of Participants (Studies)	Quality of the Evidence (GRADE)	Relative Effect (95% CI)	Anticipated Absolute Effects	
				Risk with Placebo	Risk Difference with CHM
Lung function: FEV$_1$% Treatment duration: mean 4 weeks	106 (2 RCTs)	⊕⊕⊕O MODERATE[1]	—	The mean FEV$_1$, in the control group was **70.5%**.	**MD 2.87 higher** (1.96 lower to 7.7 higher)
Asthma control: ACT[2] Treatment duration: 4 weeks	43 (1 RCT)	⊕⊕⊕O MODERATE[1]	—	The mean ACT in the control group was **16.81** points.	**MD 1.55 higher** (0.52 higher to 2.58 higher)
Lung function PEF L/s, use of rescue medication, exacerbation frequency, and quality of life — not reported					
Adverse events	None of the studies reported if adverse events occurred.				

NB. The risk in the intervention group (and its 95% CI) is based on the assumed risk in the comparison group and the relative effect of the intervention (and its 95% CI).

Abbreviations: ACT, Asthma Control Test; CHM: Chinese Herbal Medicine; CI: Confidence Interval; FEV1, Forced Effective Volume; GRADE, Grading of Recommendations Assessment, Development and Evaluation; MD: Mean Difference; RCT, Randomised Controlled Trial.

Notes:
1. Small sample size limits certainty of results
2. ACT: 5-25 points. Higher scores indicate more controlled asthma.

Study References:
▪ Lung function: H40, H65
▪ Asthma control: H40

Table 5.9 GRADE: CHM plus Pharmacotherapy vs. Pharmacotherapy for Chronic Asthma

Outcomes and Follow-up	No. of Participants (Studies)	Quality of the Evidence (GRADE)	Relative Effect (95% CI)	Risk with Pharmacotherapy	Anticipated Absolute Effects Risk Difference with CHM plus Pharmacotherapy
Lung function FEV$_1$ % Treatment duration: mean 10 weeks	2283 (21 RCTs)	⊕⊕⊕○ LOW [1,2]	—	The mean FEV$_1$ in the control group was **72.5%**	MD **7.14 higher** (5.24 higher to 9.03 higher)
Lung function PEF L/s Treatment duration: mean 6.5 weeks	1562 (14 RCTs)	⊕⊕⊕○ LOW [1,2]	—	The mean PEF in the control group was **4.39 L/s**	MD **0.83 higher** (0.47 higher to 1.19 higher)
Asthma control ACT[4] Treatment duration: mean 16 weeks	561 (5 RCTs)	⊕⊕⊕○ LOW [1,2]	—	The mean ACT in the control group was **20.12** points	MD **2.47 higher** (1.64 higher to 3.29 higher)
Use of rescue medication Puffs Treatment duration: mean 12 weeks	194 (2 RCTs)	⊕⊕○○ VERY LOW [1,2,3]	—	The mean rescue bronchodilator use in the control group was **2.53** puffs	MD **1.14 lower** (2.2 lower to 0.09 lower)
Exacerbation frequency Treatment duration: 1 year	143 (1 RCT)	⊕⊕⊕○ LOW [1,3]	—	The mean exacerbation frequency in the control group was **4.3** exacerbations	MD **1.2 lower** (1.82 lower to 0.58 lower)

(Continued)

Table 5.9 *(Continued)*

Outcomes and Follow-up	No. of Participants (Studies)	Quality of the Evidence (GRADE)	Relative Effect (95% CI)	Anticipated Absolute Effects	
				Risk with Pharmacotherapy	Risk Difference with CHM plus Pharmacotherapy
Quality of life AQLQ[5] Treatment duration: 12 weeks	142 (1 RCT)	⊕⊕○○ LOW[1,3]	—	The mean AQLQ in the control group was **154.81** points	MD **2.22 higher** (2.3 lower to 6.74 higher)
Adverse events			Adverse events were reported in four studies. Event numbers were not given but adverse events included discomfort in the throat, hoarseness and fungal infection in the throat (H103), discomfort in the stomach and abdomen (H108), fullness of the chest, cough, insomnia (H131), and hoarseness, fungal infection in the mouth, palpitation and tremor of the hand (H193).		

NB. The risk in the intervention group (and its 95% CI) is based on the assumed risk in the comparison group and the relative effect of the intervention (and its 95% CI).

Abbreviations: ACT, Asthma Control Test; AQLQ, Asthma Quality of Life Questionnaire; CHM: Chinese Herbal Medicine; CI: Confidence Interval; FEV1, Forced Effective Volume; GRADE, Grading of Recommendations Assessment, Development and Evaluation; MD: Mean Difference; RCT, Randomised Controlled Trial.

Notes:

1. Lack of blinding of participants and personnel.
2. Considerable statistical heterogeneity.
3. Small sample size limits certainty of results.
4. ACT: 5-25 points. Higher scores indicate more controlled asthma.
5. AQLQ: 32 items, range: 32-224 points. Higher scores indicate better quality of life.

Study References:

- Lung function FEV$_1$%: H81, H103, H108, H111, H124, H127, H134, H147, H151, H154, H159, H168, H174, H182, H185, H190, H191, H193, H205, H222, H243
- Lung function PEF L/s: H97, H108, H111, H124, H148, H154, H157, H163, H167, H180, H203, H211, H244, H245
- Asthma control: H99, H103, H146, H157, H204
- Use of rescue medication: H167, H205
- Exacerbation frequency: H238
- Quality of life: H248

Table 5.10 GRADE: Bu Zhong Yi Qi Tang plus Pharmacotherapy vs. Pharmacotherapy for Chronic Asthma

Outcomes and Follow-up	No. of Participants (Studies)	Quality of the Evidence (GRADE)	Relative Effect (95% CI)	Anticipated Absolute Effects	
				Risk with Pharmacotherapy	Risk Difference with Bu zhong yi qi tang plus Pharmacotherapy
Lung function FEV$_1$ % Treatment duration: 10 weeks	131 (1 RCT)	⊕⊕OO LOW[1,2]	—	The mean FEV$_1$ in the control group was **69%**	MD **4 % higher** (0.3 lower to 8.3 higher)
Lung function PEF L/s, asthma control, use of rescue medication, exacerbation frequency, and quality of life — not reported					
Adverse events	None of the studies reported if adverse events occurred.				

NB. The risk in the intervention group (and its 95% CI) is based on the assumed risk in the comparison group and the relative effect of the intervention (and its 95% CI).

Abbreviations: CHM: Chinese Herbal Medicine; CI: Confidence Interval; FEV$_1$, Forced Expiratory Volume in One Second; GRADE, Grading of Recommendations Assessment, Development and Evaluation; MD: Mean Difference; PEF, Peak Expiratory Flow; RCT, Randomised Controlled Trials.

Notes:
1. Lack of blinding of participants and personnel.
2. Small sample size limits certainty of results.

Study References:
▪ Lung function: H127

Frequently Reported Herbs in Meta-Analyses Showing Favourable Effect

The most frequently reported herbs in meta-analyses showing favourable effects were calculated according to outcome category. Commonly used herbs for lung function FEV_1, FVC, or PEF in positive meta-analysis were *gan cao* 甘草 and *ma huang* 麻黄. *Huang qi* 黄芪 and *dang shen* 党参 were commonly used for asthma control, and *ma huang* 麻黄 and *gan cao* 甘草 were commonly used for effective rate. Table 5.11 includes the full list of herbs.

Acute Exacerbations of Asthma

Lung Function

During acute exacerbations of asthma, CHM was given orally or through a nebulised inhaler. In terms of lung function, oral CHM plus pharmacotherpy improved FEV_1 by 0.31 L ([0.22, 0.39], $I^2 = 88\%$) and 6.47% ([3.90, 9.04], $I^2 = 93\%$), and FVC by 0.33 L ([0.22, 0.44], $I^2 = 33\%$) (Table 5.12). When oral CHM alone was compared with pharmacotherapies, including beta2-agonists, steroids, antibiotics, and theophylline, FEV_1 L improved MD (0.13 L ([0.02, 0.24], $I^2 = 78\%$), but FEV_1% did not improve (MD, 2.69% ([–0.02, 5.40], $I^2 = 71\%$) (Table 5.12).

Peak expiratory flow after oral CHM alone or as integrative medicine improved lung function by 0.45 L/s ([0.21, 0.69], $I^2 = 76\%$) and 0.66 L/s ([0.44, 0.88], $I^2 = 70\%$), respectively (Table 5.12). Although there were positive results, there was significant heterogeneity in the pooled results in terms of interventions, length of treatments, and severity of asthma. The frequently used herbs in positive meta-analyses were *ma huang* 麻黄, *ban xia* 半夏, *gan cao* 甘草, *xing ren* 杏仁, and *huang qin* 黄芩.

Two studies compared CHM with placebos. When *Qu chuan tang* 祛喘汤 plus pharmacotherapy was compared with a placebo and with pharmacotherapy, PEF L/s improved in one study (MD 1.01 L/s [0.57, 1.45]) (H128). One study compared *Yi qi ping chuan* granules 益气平喘颗粒 against a placebo and found no difference

Table 5.11 Frequently Reported Herbs in Meta-analyses Showing Favourable Effect for Chronic Asthma

Outcome Category	No. of Meta-analyses	No. of Studies	Herbs	Scientific Name	No. of Studies Using Herb
Lung Function (FEV₁, FVC)	7	54	Gan cao 甘草	*Glycyrrhiza spp.*	24
			Ma huang 麻黄	*Ephedra spp.*	18
			Di long 地龙	*Pheretima spp.*	14
			Huang qi 黄芪	*Astragalus membranaceus* (Fisch.) Bge.	14
			Xing ren 杏仁	*Prunus armeniaca* L.	13
			Wu wei zi 五味子	*Schisandra chinensis* (Turcz.) Baill.	13
			Fang feng 防风	*Saposhnikovia divaricata* (Turcz.) Schischk.	11
			Bai zhu 白术	*Atractylodes macrocephala* Koidz.	11
			Ban xia 半夏	*Pinellia ternata* (Thunb.) Breit.	10
			Dang gui 当归	*Angelica sinensis* (Oliv.) Diels	9
			Chen pi 陈皮	*Citrus reticulata* Blanco	8
			Dang shen 党参	*Codonopsis spp.*	8
			Yin yang huo 淫羊藿	*Epimedium spp.*	8
Lung Function (PEF)	2	23	Gan cao 甘草	*Glycyrrhiza spp.*	9
			Ma huang 麻黄	*Ephedra spp.*	9
			Ban xia 半夏	*Pinellia ternata* (Thunb.) Breit.	6
			Di long 地龙	*Pheretima spp.*	6

(Continued)

Table 5.11: (*Continued*)

Outcome Category	No. of Meta-analyses	No. of Studies	Herbs	Scientific Name	No. of Studies Using Herb
			Xing ren 杏仁	*Prunus armeniaca* L.	6
			Tao ren 桃仁	*Prunus spp.*	5
			Xi xin 细辛	*Asarum spp.*	5
			Dan shen 丹参	*Salvia miltiorrhiza* Bge.	5
			Wu wei zi 五味子	*Schisandra chinensis* (Turcz.) Baill.	5
			Huang qi 黄芪	*Astragalus membranaceus* (Fisch.) Bge.	4
			Kuan dong hua 款冬花	*Tussilago farfara* L.	4
Asthma Control (ACT)	1	5	Huang qi 黄芪	*Astragalus membranaceus* (Fisch.) Bge.	4
			Dang shen 党参	*Codonopsis spp.*	3
			Quan xie 全蝎	*Buthus martensi* Karsch	3
			Ban xia 半夏	*Pinellia ternata* (Thunb.) Breit.	2
			Chan tui 蝉蜕	*Cyptotympana atrata* Fabricius.	2
			Gan cao 甘草	*Glycyrrhiza spp.*	2
			Jiang can 僵蚕	*Bombyx mori* L.	2
			Jiang huang 姜黄	*Curcuma longa* L.	2
			Wu gong 蜈蚣	*Scolopendra subspinipes mutilans* L. Koch	2

Effective Rate	4	29			
			Ma huang 麻黄	*Ephedra spp.*	6
			Gan cao 甘草	*Glycyrrhiza spp.*	5
			Jiang can 僵蚕	*Bombyx mori* L.	5
			Di long 地龙	*Pheretima spp.*	4
			Wu wei zi 五味子	*Schisandra chinensis* (Turcz.) Baill.	4
			Chan tui 蝉蜕	*Cyptotympana atrata* Fabricius.	3
			Xing ren 杏仁	*Prunus armeniaca* L.	3
			Yin yang huo 淫羊藿	*Epimedium spp.*	3
			Zi su zi 紫苏子	*Perilla frutescens* (L.) Britt.	3

Meta-analysis references

- Lung function (FEV$_1$, FVC): CHM v. pharmacotherapy (FEV$_1$L), CHM v. pharmacotherapy (FEV$_1$%), CHM v. pharmacotherapy (FVCL), CHM v. pharmacotherapy (FVC%), CHM + pharmacotherapy v. pharmacotherapy (FEV$_1$L), CHM + pharmacotherapy v. pharmacotherapy (FEV1%), CHM + pharmacotherapy v. pharmacotherapy (FVCL)
- Lung function (PEF): CHM + pharmacotherapy v. pharmacotherapy, CHM + pharmacotherapy v. placebo + pharmacotherapy
- Asthma control: CHM + pharmacotherapy v. pharmacotherapy
- Effective rate: CHM v. pharmacotherapy (TCM Syndrome Diagnostic), CHM v. pharmacotherapy (Clinical Research Guidelines), CHM v. pharmacotherapy (Bronc. Asthma Guide), CHM + pharmacotherapy v. pharmacotherapy (Bronc. Asthma Guide)

Frequently reported herbs in meta-analyses showing favourable effect are calculated by selecting the effective pools for each outcome category based on the intervention type. The herbs used in the individual studies are then counted. Pools are considered to be effective if they show a statistically significant effect at end of treatment between groups.

Abbreviations: ACT, Asthma Control Test; CHM, Chinese Herbal Medicine; FEV$_1$, Forced Expiratory Volume in One Second; FVC, Forced Vital Capacity; TCM, Traditional Chinese Medicine; PEF, Peak Expiratory Flow.

Table 5.12   Oral CHM — Lung Function (Acute Exacerbations of Asthma)

Comparator	Outcome	No. of Studies	No. of Participants	Effect Size MD [95% CI]	I^2 %	Included Studies
Pharmacotherapy	FEV$_1$ L	12	983	0.13 [0.02, 0.24]*	78	H12, H23, H25, H26, H34, H36–H38, H43, H49, H68, H79
Pharmacotherapy	FEV$_1$ %	6	711	2.69 [–0.02, 5.40]	71	H12, H15, H20, H49, H64, H77
Pharmacotherapy	FVC L	4	381	0.17 [–0.00, 0.33]	68	H12, H36, H38, H79
Pharmacotherapy	PEF L/s	9	741	0.45 [0.21, 0.69]*	76	H12, H25, H34, H36, H37, H38, H43, H68, H79
Integrative medicine	FEV$_1$ L	30	2290	0.31 [0.22, 0.39]*	88	H83, H96, H101, H106, H109, H110, H112, H116, H117, H120, H121, H122, H123, H125, H136, H137, H140, H153, H164, H171, H179, H189, H198, H202, H210, H212, H221, H226, H228, H230, H231
Integrative medicine	FEV$_1$ %	20	1708	6.47 [3.90, 9.04]*	93	H83, H90, H96, H98, H109, H112, H116, H123, H136, H150, H153, H170, H179, H212, H221, H223, H228, H234, H242
Integrative medicine	FVC L	8	620	0.33 [0.22, 0.44]*	33	H96, H116, H121, H125, H210, H221, H228, H230
Integrative medicine	PEF L/s	16	1251	0.66 [0.44, 0.88]*	70	H106, H110, H112, H116, H117, H121, H122, H125, H137, H142, H179, H198, H202, H210, H228, H231

*Statistically significant
Abbreviations: CI, Confidence Interval; CHM, Chinese Herbal Medicine; FEV$_1$, Forced Expiratory Volume in One Second; FVC, Forced Vital Capacity; MD, Mean Difference; PEF, Peak Expiratory Flow.

between the CHM and control group in terms of PEF (MD 0.43 L/s [−0.46, 1.32]) (H240).

Health-related Quality of Life

Health-related quality of life was not evaluated in any of the studies.

Asthma Control

The ACT was administered to participants and evaluated in four studies. Asthma control improved after CHM plus pharmacotherapy compared with pharmacotherapy alone by 3.11 points ([1.27, 4.94], $I^2 = 93\%$) (H107, H117, H121, H242).

Use of Rescue Medication

The use of rescue medication was evaluated in one study. Results showed that *Jia jian wu mei wan* 加减乌梅丸 plus corticosteroids (budesonide) compared with budesonide alone did not significantly reduce salbutamol usage (MD −0.04 puffs [−0.50, 0.42]) (H231).

Effective Rate

Most studies evaluated investigator-rated symptoms of asthma, which serves as the measure of effective rate. The three main guidelines used in the studies were the TCM Syndrome Diagnostic Efficacy Standards, the CM Clinical Research Guidelines, and the Bronchial Asthma Guide. Combined with pharmacotherapy, CHM improved asthma symptoms based on all guidelines (Table 5.13). The largest result was seen on the TCM Syndrome Diagnostic Efficacy Standards, where the chance of achieving improvement in symptoms with CHM was 1.21 that of the control group ([1.08, 1.35]; $I^2 = 51\%$) (Table 5.13).

Alone, CHM improved the effective based on the Bronchial Asthma Guide by 1.16 times that of control [1.02, 1.31]; $I^2 = 72\%$) (Table 5.13). However, studies were heterogeneous and sub-group analysis did not reduce heterogeneity, therefore limiting the certainty

Table 5.13   Oral CHM — Effective Rate (Acute Exacerbations of Asthma)

Comparator	Outcome	No. of Studies	No. of Participants	Effect Size RR [95% CI]	I² %	Included Studies
Pharmacotherapy	Bronchial Asthma Guide	6	739	1.16 [1.02, 1.31]*	72	H18, H20, H37, H41, H70, H246
Pharmacotherapy	CM Clinical Research Guidelines	5	474	1.06 [0.98, 1.14]	54	H25, H34, H38, H64, H68
Integrative medicine	Bronchial Asthma Guide	31	2453	1.15 [1.10, 1.20]*	56	H83, H84, H88, H89, H90, H98, H101, H109, H118, H120, H121, H122, H123, H130, H136, H140, H141, H142, H153, H162, H171, H172, H186, H188, H196, H197, H210, H215, H232, H234, H246
Integrative medicine	CM Clinical Research Guidelines	9	685	1.14 [1.05, 1.24]*	55	H86, H106, H117, H126, H137, H150, H164, H230, H242
Integrative medicine	TCM Syndrome Diagnostic Efficacy Standards	4	564	1.21 [1.08, 1.35]*	51	H81, H109, H143, H233

*Statistically significant

Abbreviations: CI, Confidence Interval; CHM, Chinese Herbal Medicine; TCM, Traditional Chinese Medicine; CM, Chinese Medicine; RR, Risk Ratio.

of results. The frequently used herbs in positive meta-analyses were *ma huang* 麻黄, *gan cao* 甘草, *ban xia* 半夏, *xing ren* 杏仁, and *wu wei zi* 五味子. Studies that used the CM Clinical Research Guidelines did not show statistical differences between CHM and controls (Table 5.13).

Assessment Using GRADE: Acute Exacerbations of Asthma

The main comparison for acute exacerbations of asthma is presented in a GRADE summary of findings table. The quality of the evidence for CHM plus pharmacotherapy compared to pharmacotherapy alone was between very low and low (Table 5.14). The result was statistically significant for $FEV_1\%$ and PEF L/s. Asthma control was not statistically significant.

Randomised Controlled Trial Evidence from Individual Formula and Formula Commonly Used in Clinical Practice

Four formulae, *Xiao qing long tang* 小青龙汤, *She gan ma huang tang* 射干麻黄汤, *Ding chuan tang* 定喘汤, and *Ma xing shi gan tang* 麻杏石甘汤, were used in multiple clinical trials. *Xiao qing long tang* 小青龙汤 and *Ma xing shi gan tang* 麻杏石甘汤 were evaluated in meta-analyses. Studies evaluating *She gan ma huang tang* 射干麻黄汤 and *Ding chuan tang* 定喘汤 evaluated different outcomes and could not be pooled for analysis.

Xiao qing long tang 小青龙汤 plus pharmacotherapy improved the effective rate based on the Bronchial Asthma Guide by 1.18 times that of pharmacotherapy alone ([1.05, 1.32]; $I^2 = 0\%$) (Table 5.15). *Ma xing shi gan tang* 麻杏石甘汤 plus pharmacotherapy also improved the effective rate similarly to *Xiao qing long tang* based on the TCM Syndrome Diagnostic Efficacy Standards, where the chance of achieving improvement in symptoms with CHM was 1.20 times that of pharmacotherapy alone ([1.04, 1.38]; $I^2 = 0\%$). *Ma xing shi gan tang* 麻杏石甘汤 plus pharmacotherapy also improved $FEV_1\%$ by 8.30% compared to pharmacotherapy alone ([2.06, 14.53]; $I^2 = 82\%$) (Table 5.15).

Table 5.14 GRADE: CHM plus Pharmacotherapy vs. Pharmacotherapy for Acute Exacerbations of Asthma

Outcomes and Follow-up	No. of Participants (Studies)	Quality of the Evidence (GRADE)	Relative Effect (95% CI)	Anticipated Absolute Effects	
				Risk with Pharmacotherapy	Risk difference with CHM plus Pharmacotherapy
Lung function FEV$_1$ % Treatment duration: mean 4.75 weeks	1708 (20 RCTs)	⊕⊕◯◯ LOW[1,2]	—	The mean FEV$_1$ in the control group was 77.9 %	MD 6.47 **higher** (3.90 higher to 9.04 higher)
Lung function PEF L/s Treatment duration: mean 3.8 weeks	1251 (16 RCTs)	⊕⊕◯◯ LOW[1,2]	—	The mean PEF in the control group was **5.6 L/s**	MD 0.66 **higher** (0.44 higher to 0.88 higher)
Asthma control ACT[5] Treatment duration: mean 9.5 weeks	281 (4 RCTs)	⊕◯◯◯ VERY LOW[1,2,3]	—	The mean ACT in the control group was **23.8** points	MD 3.11 **higher** (1.27 higher to 4.94 higher)
Use of rescue medication Puffs Treatment duration: 12 weeks	40 (1 RCT)	⊕⊕◯◯ LOW[1,3]	—	The mean rescue bronchodilator use in the control group was **2.8** puffs	MD 0.04 **lower** (0.5 lower to 0.42 higher)

Adverse events

Eleven studies reported adverse events. Six of the studies reported that no events occurred (H114, H126, H164, H199, H202, H242). Seven studies reported adverse events including fullness and discomfort in the abdomen, skin rash, nausea, vomiting, headache, palpitations, pricking pain in the throat, discomfort of the throat and hoarseness. Adverse events in the control groups were similar and also included insomnia and increased heart rate (H85, H121, H150, H171, H183, H189, H230)

NB. The risk in the intervention group (and its 95% CI) is based on the assumed risk in the comparison group and the relative effect of the intervention (and its 95% CI).

Abbreviations: ACT, Asthma Control Test; CI, Confidence Interval; CHM, Chinese Herbal Medicine; FEV_1, Forced Expiratory Volume in One Second; GRADE, Grading of Recommendations Assessment, Development and Evaluation; RCT, Randomised Controlled Trial; MD, Mean Difference; PEF, Peak Expiratory Flow.

Notes:

1. Lack of blinding of participants and personnel.
2. Considerable statistical heterogeneity.
3. Small sample size limits certainty of results.
4. ACT: 5-25 points. Higher scores indicate more controlled asthma.

Study References:

- Lung function (FEV1%): H83, H90, H96, H98, H109, H112, H116, H123, H136, H142, H150, H153, H170, H179, H212, H221, H223, H228, H234, H242
- Lung function (PEF L/s): H106, H110, H112, H116, H117, H121, H122, H125, H137, H142, H179, H198, H202, H210, H228, H231
- Asthma control: H110, H117, H121, H242
- Use of rescue medication: H231

Table 5.15. Lung Function — Effective Rate (Individual Formula)

Intervention	Comparator	Outcome	No. of Studies	No. of Participants	Effect Size MD/RR [95% CI]	I² %	Included Studies
Xiao qing long tang 小青龙汤	Integrative medicine	Bronchial Asthma Guide	2	147	1.18 [1.05, 1.32]*	0	H130, H215
Ma xing shi gan tang 麻杏石甘汤	Integrative medicine	FEV₁ %	2	120	8.30 [2.06, 14.53]*	82	H98, H136
		TCM Syndrome Diagnostic Efficacy Standards	2	120	1.20 [1.04, 1.38]*	0	H98, H136
She gan ma huang tang 射干麻黄汤	Integrative medicine	FEV₁ L	2	147	0.82 [0.52, 1.11]*	33	H117, H123
		Bronchial Asthma Guide	2	168	1.20 [1.06, 1.36]*	0	H123, H232

*Statistically significant

Abbreviations: CI, Confidence Interval; FEV_1, Forced Expiratory Volume in One Second; MD, Mean Difference; RR, Risk Ratio; TCM, Traditional Chinese Medicine.

Compared to pharmacotherapy alone, *She gan ma huang tang* 射干麻黄汤 was found to improve FEV_1 by 0.82 L ([0.52, 1.11]; $I^2 = 33\%$) and the effective rate (based on the Bronchial Asthma Guide) by 1.20 times ([1.06, 1.36]; $I^2 = 0\%$) (Table 5.15).

Assessment Using GRADE

The main comparison for acute exacerbations of asthma is presented in a GRADE summary of findings table. *Xiao qing long tang* 小青龙汤, *She gan ma huang tang* 射干麻黄汤, and *Ding chuan tang* 定喘汤 could not be included because studies did not report any of the predefined outcomes. The quality of evidence for *Ma xing shi gan tang* 麻杏石甘汤 plus pharmacotherapy compared to pharmacotherapy alone was very low (Table 5.16). The result was statistically significant for $FEV_1\%$. Other outcomes were not reported.

Table 5.16   GRADE: Ma Xing Shi Gan Tang 麻杏石甘汤 plus Pharmacotherapy vs. Pharmacotherapy for Acute Exacerbations of Asthma

Outcomes and Follow-up	No. of Participants (Studies)	Quality of the Evidence (GRADE)	Relative Effect (95% CI)	Anticipated Absolute Effects	
				Risk with Pharmacotherapy	Risk Difference with Ma xing shi gan tang plus Pharmacotherapy
Lung function FEV$_1$ % Treatment duration: mean 11 days	120 (2 RCTs)	⊕○○○ VERY LOW [1,2,3]	—	The mean FEV$_1$ % was **68.4** %	MD **8.3** % **higher** (2.06 higher to 14.53 higher)
Lung function PEF L/s, asthma control, use of rescue medication, and quality of life — not reported					
Adverse events	None of the studies reported if adverse events occurred.				

*The risk in the intervention group (and its 95% CI) is based on the assumed risk in the comparison group and the relative effect of the intervention (and its 95% CI).

Abbreviations: CI, Confidence Interval; FEV$_1$, Forced Expiratory Volume in One Second; GRADE, Grading of Recommendations Assessment, Development and Evaluation; RCT, Randomised Controlled Trial; MD, Mean Difference; PEF, Peak Expiratory Flow.

Notes:

1. Lack of blinding of participants and personnel.
2. Considerable statistical heterogeneity.
3. Small sample size limits certainty of results.

Study References:

• Lung function: H98, H136

Table 5.17 Frequently Reported Herbs in Meta-analyses Showing Favourable Effect for Acute Exacerbations of Asthma

Outcome Category	No. of Meta-analyses	No. of Studies	Herbs	Scientific Name	No. of Studies Using Herb
Lung function (FEV₁, FVC)	4	44	Ma huang 麻黄	*Ephedra spp.*	30
			Gan cao 甘草	*Glycyrrhiza spp.*	23
			Ban xia 半夏	*Pinellia ternata* (Thunb.) Breit.	22
			Xing ren 杏仁	*Prunus armeniaca* L.	22
			Huang qin 黄芩	*Scutellaria baicalensis* Georgi	18
			Di long 地龙	*Pheretima spp.*	16
			Zi su zi 紫苏子	*Perilla frutescens* (L.) Britt.	15
			Wu wei zi 五味子	*Schisandra chinensis* (Turcz.) Baill.	13
			Chen pi 陈皮	*Citrus reticulata* Blanco	12
			Tao ren 桃仁	*Prunus spp.*	10
			Xi xin 细辛	*Asarum spp.*	10
Lung function (PEF)	5	33	Ma huang 麻黄	*Ephedra spp.*	24
			Gan cao 甘草	*Glycyrrhiza spp.*	19
			Ban xia 半夏	*Pinellia ternata* (Thunb.) Breit.	18
			Huang qin 黄芩	*Scutellaria baicalensis* Georgi	17
			Di long 地龙	*Pheretima spp.*	16
			Xing ren 杏仁	*Prunus armeniaca* L.	16
			Xi xin 细辛	*Asarum spp.*	11
			Zi su zi 紫苏子	*Perilla frutescens* (L.) Britt.	11
			She gan 射干	*Belamcanda chinensis* (L.) DC.	9
			Wu wei zi 五味子	*Schisandra chinensis* (Turcz.) Baill.	8

Effective rate	5	51			
			Ma huang 麻黄	*Ephedra spp.*	34
			Gan cao 甘草	*Glycyrrhiza spp.*	28
			Ban xia 半夏	*Pinellia ternata* (Thunb.) Breit.	26
			Xing ren 杏仁	*Prunus armeniaca* L.	22
			Wu wei zi 五味子	*Schisandra chinensis* (Turcz.) Baill.	18
			Zi su zi 紫苏子	*Perilla frutescens* (L.) Britt.	15
			Di long 地龙	*Pheretima spp.*	14
			Chen pi 陈皮	*Citrus tangerina* Hort.et Tanaka	12
			Xi xin 细辛	*Asarum spp.*	12
			Bai shao 白芍	*Paeonia lactiflora* Pall.	11
			Huang qin 黄芩	*Scutellaria baicalensis* Georgi	11
			Kuan dong hua 款冬花	*Tussilago farfara* L.	11

Meta-analysis references

- Lung function (FEV$_1$, FVC): CHM v. parmacotherapy (FEV$_1$L), CHM + parmacotherapy v. parmacotherapy (FEV$_1$L), CHM + parmacotherapy v. parmacotherapy (FEV$_1$%), CHM + parmacotherapy v. parmacotherapy (FVCL)
- Lung function (PEF): CHM v. parmacotherapy (L/s), CHM + parmacotherapy v. parmacotherapy (L/s), CHM + parmacotherapy v. parmacotherapy (mL/s), CHM + parmacotherapy v. parmacotherapy (%), CHM + parmacotherapy v. parmacotherapy (variability)
- Effective rate: CHM v. parmacotherapy (TCM Syndrome), CHM v. parmacotherapy (Bronc. Asthma Guide), CHM + parmacotherapy v. parmacotherapy (TCM Syndrome), CHM + parmacotherapy v. parmacotherapy (Clinical Research Guidelines), CHM + parmacotherapy v. parmacotherapy (Bronc. Asthma Guide)

Frequently reported herbs in meta-analyses showing favourable effect are calculated by selecting the effective pools for each outcome category based on the intervention type. The herbs used in the individual studies are then counted. Pools are considered to be effective if they show a statistically significant effect at end of treatment between groups.

Abbreviations: CHM, Chinese Herbal Medicine; FEV$_1$, Forced Expiratory Volume in One Second; FVC, Forced Vital Capacity; PEF, Peak Expiratory Flow; TCM, Traditional Chinese Medicine.

Frequently Reported Herbs in Meta-Analyses Showing Favourable Effect

The most frequently reported herbs in meta-analyses showing favourable effects were calculated according to each outcome category. Commonly used herbs for lung function FEV_1 and FVC were *ma huang* 麻黄 and *xing ren* 杏仁. *Ma huang* 麻黄 and *gan cao* 甘草 were most commonly used in studies assessing effective rate. Table 5.17 includes the full list of herbs.

Safety of Chinese Herbal Medicine in Randomised Controlled Trials

Adverse events were reported in 43 studies (17.5%). Twenty-two studies stated that no events occurred (H23,H26, H42, H52,H53, H79, H114, H126, H134, H36, H146, H154, H159, H164, H180, H185, H199, H202, H203, H221, H224, H242). In the remaining 21 studies (H5, H8, H9, H34, H44, H45,H66, H78, H85, H103, H108, H121, H131, H150, H171,H183, H189, H193, H230, H239, H241), one study did not specify the nature of the adverse event (H239), while another reported an unspecified number of cases of throat discomfort (H230). Both studies were excluded from further analysis.

In the 19 studies, 66 adverse events were reported in the CHM groups, and 146 adverse events in the comparator groups. Adverse events among people who received CHM included 15 cases of fullness/discomfort in the abdoment/stomach, seven cases of nausea, six cases each of throat discomfort and fullness of the chest, five cases of hoarseness, four cases of stomach discomfort, three cases each of fungal infection in the oral cavity or throat, hand tremor, irritable cough, and palpitations, two cases of constipation, two cases of dental ulcer, and one cases each of headache, sensation of heat on the palms, insomnia, mild sinus tachycardia, nausea and fullness/discomfort in the stomach, skin rash, and vomiting

In the comparator groups, adverse events included 16 cases of hoarse voice, 15 cases of insomnia, 14 cases of stomach discomfort, 11 cases of nausea, 11 cases of throat discomfort,11 cases of palpitations, nine cases of hand tremor, eight cases of muscle tremor, agitation and insomnia, seven cases of fungal infection in the oral cavity or throat, six cases of nausea, vomiting and poor appetite, five cases of dry and painful throat, four cases each of agitation, fullness/discomfort in the stomach/abdomen, high blood pressure, and skin rash, three cases of palpitation and headache, three cases of vomiting, two cases of arrhythmia, two cases of dry mouth, two cases of fullness in the abdomen with poor appetite, two cases of fullness in the chest with palpitations, two cases of irritable cough and one case of headache.

Adverse events such as dry mouth and throat, hoarseness, and fungal infection in the throat are known side effect of steroid medication. In the studies that reported these adverse events, inhaled steroids were used. In one study using a nebulised inhalation of Yin xin nei zhi (银杏内), six participants complained of fullness of the chest in the intervention group and control group; two participants in each group out because of the fullness of the chest (H131). In the two studies reporting poor appetite, headache, nausea, fullness in the abdomen, palpitation, and insomnia events occurred in the control groups taking theophylline; no events were reported in the intervention groups of these two studies (H45, H66). Overall, CHM was well tolerated and is safe for adults with asthma.

Controlled Clinical Trials of Chinese Herbal Medicine

CHM was evaluated in 18 non-randomised controlled clinical trials (2,151 participants) (H247–H264). Six studies evaluated chronic asthma (H247–H252) and 12 evaluated acute exacerbations of asthma (H253–2H64).

CHM treatments were diverse and none of the formulae were used in more than one study. Oral herbs were the main form of administration in all studies except for one that used a nebulised inhaler. A total of 75 different herbs were used and the most common were *ma huang* 麻黄, *gan cao* 甘草, *xing ren* 杏仁, *wu wei zi* 五味子, *di long* 地龙, *huang qi* 黄芪, and *ban xia* 半夏. Comparators included pharmacotherapy in all studies except one that compared

CHM to no treatment. CHM plus pharmacotherapy compared to pharmacotherapy alone was evaluated in 10 studies.

Duration of asthma ranged from 16 months to 20 years and participants' age ranged from 20 to 75 years. There were 867 male and 584 female participants (the sex of 700 participants was not stated). CM syndromes were described in two studies, and these included Spleen and Kidney deficiency (H256) and phlegm-cold (H261).

Lung Function

Studies evaluating chronic asthma could not be pooled in a meta-analysis. In single studies, *Bu fei tang* 补肺汤 plus pharmacotherapy improved $FEV_1\%$ in chronic asthma (MD 8.22% [1.66, 14.78]) (H252) and in acute exacerbations of asthma (MD 10.75% [6.57, 14.93] (H255). When the use of *Ping chuan tang* 平喘汤 was compared with no treatment, lung function $FEV_1\%$ did not improve (MD −2.23% [−10.57, 6.11]) (H248).

In two studies evaluating acute exacerbations of asthma comparing CHM plus pharmacotherapy with pharmacotherapy alone, $FEV_1\%$ improved by 11.06% ([7.44, 14.68]; $I^2 = 0\%$) (Table 5.18). Peak expiratory flow was evaluated in three acute asthma studies (H255, H256, H259), and PEF was found to increase by 0.26 L/s after treatment with CHM plus pharmacotherapy ([0.09, 0.42]; $I^2 = 0\%$) (Table 5.18).

Health-related Quality of Life

Health-related quality of life was not evaluated in any of the studies.

Asthma Control

Participants completed the ACT in one study to determine if there are any differences in asthma control when comparing modified *Qi wei du qi wan* combined with *Liu jun zi tang* 七味都气丸合六君子汤 plus fluticasone/salmeterol to fluticasone/salmeterol alone. Compared to the control group, asthma control was better in the intervention group by 1.48 points ([0.22, 2.74]) H256.

Table 5.18   Oral CHM — Lung Function (Controlled clinical Trials)

Asthma Stage	Comparator	Outcome	No. of Studies	No. of Participants	Effect Size MD [95% CI]	I^2 %	Included Studies
Acute	Integrative medicine	FEV$_1$ %	2	150	11.06 [7.44, 14.68]*	0	H255, H259
Acute	Integrative medicine	PEF L/s	3	214	0.26 [0.09, 0.42]*	0	H255, H256, H259

*Statistically significant

Abbreviations: CHM, Chinese Herbal Medicine; CI, Confidence Interval; FEV$_1$, Forced Expiratory Volume in One Second; MD, Mean Difference; PEF, Peak Expiratory Flow.

Use of Rescue Medication

The use of rescue medication was not evaluated in any of the studies.

Effective Rate

The Bronchial Asthma Guide was used in three studies investigating acute exacerbations of asthma. The effective rate among those who received CHM plus pharmacotherapy was 1.16 that of pharmaco-therapy alone ([1.08, 1.25]; I^2 = 0%) (H254, H262, H264).

The Chinese Medicine Clinical Research Guideline was used in two studies; however, results could not be pooled (H249, H261). In one study, formulae based on syndromes combined with pharmaco-therapy were found to improve the effective rate by 1.27 times that of aminophylline for chronic asthma [1.04, 1.54] (H249). In the other study, the effective rate with CHM as integrative medicine was not statistically different to pharmacotherapy (RR 1.22 [0.98, 1.52])

Safety of Chinese Herbal Medicine in Controlled Clinical Trials

Adverse events were reported in two non-randomised controlled trials (11.1%) (H252, H256). One study reported that no events occurred (H256) and one reported a total of eight adverse events (H252). Dry mouth was reported in four people after taking *Bu fei tang* 补肺汤, and in the control group taking pharmacotherapy, there were three reports of insomnia and one of abdominal distension (H252).

Non-controlled Studies of Chinese Herbal Medicine

A total of 69 case series consisting of 3,770 participants met the eligibility criteria for inclusion (H265–H333). Characteristics of the non-controlled studies were evaluated but their findings were not evaluated due to the high number of RCTs contributing better quality evidence. CM syndromes were reported in 21 studies and common syndromes were phlegm-cold or phlegm-heat, Lung and Kidney deficiency, and phlegm obstructing the Lung. Herbal decoction was commonly used in 58 studies, granules in four studies, capsules or tablets in three studies, syrup in two studies, and an oral paste in two studies. Forms of CHM were diverse, and only four formulae were used in two or more studies. The most common formula was *Ding chuan tang* 定喘汤 (four studies). A total of 159 distinct herbs were used in these studies and the most common were *ma huang* 麻黄 (43 studies), *gan cao* 甘草 (32 studies), *ban xia* 半夏 (29 studies), *xing ren* 杏仁 (27 studies), *chen pi* 陈皮 (18 studies), and *di long* 地龙 (18 studies).

Safety of Chinese Herbal Medicine in Non-controlled Studies

Adverse events were reported in seven studies (H268, H292, H298, H302, H325, H332, H333). Four studies reported that no adverse events occurred and events in the other studies were reportedly mild. Adverse events included dizziness (three cases), chest fullness, nausea, headache, and sweating (number of cases not specified). After taking a purified extract of *xin yi hua* 辛荑花, 103 adverse events were reported in 52 patients, of which 29 were classified as 'probably' or 'possibly' associated with treatment. These 29 events included indigestion (seven cases), epigastric soreness (four cases), nausea (four cases), constipation (two cases), and one case each of vomiting, abdominal pain, dysphagia, paraesthesia, migraine, facial swelling, pruritus, urticaria, rash, skin exfoliation, myalgia, and dyspnoea.

Summary of Chinese Herbal Medicine Clinical Evidence

Over 200 RCTs consisting of more than 27,000 participants were analysed. Common CM syndromes included Lung, Spleen, and Kidney deficiency, phlegm obstruction of the Lung, and phlegm-cold or phlegm-heat. CHM alone or combined with pharmacotherapy improved chronic asthma in terms of lung function (FEV_1 and PEF), asthma control, and overall effective rate based on the Bronchial Asthma Guide, the TCM Syndrome Diagnostic Efficacy Standards, and the CM Clinical Research Guidelines. In single studies, CHM also reduced exacerbation frequency and reduced the use of rescue medication (salbutamol). CHM did not improve health-related quality of life, but insufficient studies evaluated this outcome. Of the individual formulae, *Bu zhong yi qi tang* 补中益气汤 was common among studies and was found to improve lung function. *Ma huang* 麻黄 and *gan cao* 甘草 were the most commonly used herbs in formulae reporting positive results for lung function, asthma control, and effective rate. CHM appeared to be safe for chronic asthma.

During acute exacerbations of asthma, CHM improved lung function (FEV_1 and PEF) compared to pharmacotherapy. However, there was no difference between CHM and a placebo in one study. Effective rate was improved during exacerbations but there was no difference between CHM and control groups for asthma control and rescue medication. The effects of CHM on health-related quality of life were not reported in any of the acute exacerbation studies. *Xiao qing long tang* 小青龙汤 and *Ma xing shi gan tang* 麻杏石甘汤 showed improvements in effective rate but only *Ma xing shi gan tang*

麻杏石甘汤 improved lung function. *Ma huang* 麻黄, *gan cao* 甘草, *ban xia* 半夏, *xing ren* 杏仁, and *chen pi* 陈皮 were commonly used herbs in formulae reporting positive results for lung function and effective rate. Adverse events were reported; however, they were mild and similar between intervention and control groups.

While the results are generally positive, statistical heterogeneity was present which potentially reduces confidence in some of the results. Sub-group analysis was performed but it did not reduce heterogeneity. The results also showed that a broad range of CHM formulae and herbs have been used to treat asthma. The most common formulae were *Xiao qing long tang* 小青龙汤, *Ding chuan tang* 定喘汤, and *She gan ma huang tang* 射干麻黄汤 and the most common herbs were *ma huang* 麻黄, *gan cao* 甘草, *xing ren* 杏仁, and *ban xia* 半夏.

The current analysis suggests that CHM, either alone or when combined with pharmacotherapy, improves acute and chronic asthma in terms of lung function, asthma control, and effective rate. Results for other outcomes such as health-related quality of life, exacerbation frequency, and rescue medications were few in number but the current results are promising. The GRADE scale showed that the quality of evidence provided by the studies in this analysis were rather low, with the exception of CHM versus placebo studies which provided evidence of moderate quality. The included studies were at some risk of bias due to blinding, method of random sequence generation, and concealment inadequacies. Only a small number of adverse events were reported. They were considerably mild and included headache, nausea, and gastrointestinal upset. Overall, CHM appears beneficial and well tolerated for the treatment of adult asthma.

The available evidence indicates that CHM can be considered as a beneficial and safe therapeutic option for treating adult asthma. Frequently used herbs in studies reporting positive effects included *ma huang* 麻黄, *ban xia* 半夏, *wu wei zi* 五味子, *gan cao* 甘草, and *huang qi* 黄芪, and for acute exacerbations, *huang qin* 黄芩 was frequently used. CHM can be used alone or in combination with pharmacotherapies to help improve clinical outcomes such as lung function, asthma control, and overall symptom management.

References

1. Huntley A, Ernst E. Herbal medicines for asthma: A systematic review. Thorax. 2000;**55**(11):925–929.

2. Arnold E, Clark CE, Lasserson TJ, Wu T. Herbal interventions for chronic asthma in adults and children. Cochrane Database Syst Rev. 2008;**23**(1):CD005989.

3. Hong ML, Song Y, Li XM. Effects and mechanisms of actions of Chinese herbal medicines for asthma. Chin J Integr Med. 2011;**17**(7):483–91.

4. Zhen XY. (2002) Guiding Principle of Clinical Research on New Drugs of Traditional Chinese Medicine. Chinese medical science and technology press. [In Chinese: 郑筱萸. 中药新药临床研究指导原则. 中国医药科技出版社].

5. 中华人民共和国中医药行业标准. 国家中医药管理局发布. 中医病证诊断疗效标准. 1994.

6. Prevention and treatment of asthma guideline. Chin J Tuberc Respir Dis, 1997;**20**(5):261–267 [In Chinese: 支气管哮喘防治指南. 中华结核和呼吸杂志, 1997;**20**(5):261–267].

7. Schatz M, Kosinski M, Yarlas AS, Hanlon J, Watson ME, Jhingran P. The minimally important difference of the Asthma Control Test. J Allergy Clin Immunol 2009;**124**:719–23.

8. Juniper EF, Guyatt GH, Willan A, Griffith LE. Determining a minimal important change in a disease-specific quality of life questionnaire. J Clin Epidemiol 1994;**47**(1): 81–87.

References to Included Chinese Herbal Medicine Studies

Study No.	References
H1	褚东宁, 俞定珍. 虫子抗敏煎对螨性哮喘肺功能影响. 浙江中西医结合杂志. 2002,12(12):743–744
H2	赵贵铭. "培本平喘散" 治疗哮喘 108 例的临床观察. 中医药研究. 1996,6:13–14
H3	袁尚红, 任雅芳, 刘银平. 培元固本纳气汤治疗支气管哮喘 43 例. 江西中医药. 2012,43(356):19–20

(Continued)

(Continued)

Study No.	References
H4	许有慧, 牛晓亚. 利肺片治疗支气管哮喘慢性持续期 49 例. 中医杂志. 2011,52(24):2135–2136
H5	邹金盎, 顾凤琴, 廖文军, 等. 温阳通络合剂治疗寒性哮喘的临床研究. 中国中西医结合杂志. 1996,16(9):529–532
H6	朱越. 定喘汤加减治疗热性哮喘对照临床观察. 实用中医内科杂志. 2012,26(10):32–33
H7	朱晓霞. 中药平喘药在哮喘治疗中的影响探究. 中国民族民间医药杂志. 2013,22(15): 99–100
H8	朱慧志, 韩明向, 梅晓冬. 金泰冲剂治疗支气管哮喘的临床研究. 安徽中医学院学报. 2004,23(4):11–14
H9	郑翠娥, 曲政军. 喘舒颗粒治疗支气管哮喘缓解期 40 例临床观察. 山东中医药大学学报. 2003,27(3):183–184
H10	张中亮. 小青龙汤治疗支气管哮喘临床观察. 中国中医药咨讯. 2009,1(2):161
H11	张鑫, 朴宇, 郑明昱. 鹿茸大补汤对太阴人哮喘缓解期的疗效. 长春中医药大学学报. 2013,29(5):871–872
H12	张京. 蛇蝉小青龙合剂治疗寒哮临床研究. 中国中医急症. 2004,13(7):426–427
H13	张芬兰, 俞璆颖. 清肺平喘汤治疗支气管哮喘 60 例临床观察. 长春中医药大学学报. 2009,25(5):705–706
H14	张晨霞. 清热喘康方治疗支气管哮喘临床观察. 中国中医急症. 2010,19(8):1286,1302
H15	曾宪兰, 黄树红, 张振荣. 射干麻黄汤对哮喘患者血清IgE,EOS 调节的观察与分析. 临床肺科杂志. 2010,15(4):589
H16	余传星, 严桂珍, 林晶. 藿香正气口服液超声携氧雾化吸入治疗支气管哮喘发作期 42 例疗效观察. 福建中医学院学报. 2005,15(5):3–5
H17	杨继兵, 曹方会, 陈黎, 等. 芩黄合剂雾化吸入对支气管哮喘气道慢性炎症的影响. 中国中医药信息杂志. 2008,15(2):9–11
H18	杨桦, 洪杰斐, 袁汉饶. 小青龙汤对哮喘病人嗜酸性粒细胞及白介素5的影响. 辽宁中医杂志. 2004,31(6): 486–487
H19	武煦峰, 薛博瑜. 疏肝理气法治疗哮喘缓解期气道高反应性 42 例临床观察. 中医药导报. 2011,17(4):27–28
H20	吴银根, 于素霞, 张惠勇, 等. 咳喘落治疗 175 例哮喘临床总结. 上海中医药杂志. 2000,(9):19–21

(Continued)

(Continued)

Study No.	References
H21	巫建龙, 王大海, 曹伟云, 等. 补肾温肺胶囊治疗支气管哮喘 46 例临床观察. 国际医药卫生导报. 2008,14(15):94–96
H22	王文富,刘生海.止咳救肺汤治疗29例支气管哮喘临床观察.内蒙古中医药.2011,30(10): 32
H23	王历敬, 吕晓芳. 解痉止喘液雾化吸入治疗支气管哮喘疗效观察. 湖北中医杂志. 2003,25(11):25–26
H24	王建利. 中医治疗支气管哮喘患者的临床疗效分析. 中国现代药物应用. 2013,7(17):147–148
H25	王宏献. 平喘降气汤治疗支气管哮喘急性发作的临床研究. 中华中医药学刊. 2008,26(5):1114–1115
H26	王宏长, 张金福, 许峰, 等. 咳喘落对哮喘患者嗜酸性粒细胞阳离子蛋白的影响. 上海中医药杂志. 2000,34(3): 16–18
H27	汪明星. 中西医结合治疗老年轻中度慢性持续期哮喘临床效果分析. 当代医学. 2013,19(21):152–153
H28	唐兴荣, 李达仁, 谭金华. 镇喘颗粒对支气管哮喘患者神经生长因子及嗜酸性粒细胞的影响. 中医药导报. 2005,11(8):10–11,25
H29	孙航成, 谌晓莉, 朱启勇, 等. 利肺片治疗支气管哮喘(肺肾两虚证) 30 例临床观察. 长春中医药大学学报. 2012,28(2):313–314
H30	任国英. 益气平喘汤治疗支气管哮喘(缓解期)临证研究. 实用中医内科杂志. 2008,22(2):23–24
H31	马进, 乔铁, 乔世举. 固本止咳平喘颗粒治疗支气管哮喘 30 例临床研究. 云南中医中药杂志. 2011,32(4): 15–16
H32	罗祥顺, 曾华芳. 金匮肾气丸加味治疗支气管哮喘缓解期 36 例临床观察. 中医药导报. 2013,19(2):65–67
H33	刘自力, 吴兆利. 培土生金法治疗支气管哮喘(缓解期) 35 例临床观察. 中医药导报. 2006,12(1):37–38
H34	刘兰萍, 张慧琪, 刘曼. 清肺平喘汤治疗支气管哮喘发作期临床观察. 中国中医急症. 2005,14(12):1162,1164
H35	刘贵颖, 张蕴卓, 王昭杰, 等.咳喘胶囊治疗支气管哮喘慢性持续期 15 例临床观察. 中医杂志. 2008,49(7):611–613
H36	刘贵颖, 吕英, 朱振刚, 等. 咳喘口服液治疗支气管哮喘的临床研究. 天津中医药. 2004,21(3):199–201

(Continued)

Study No.	References
H37	林丹曦. 蛤蚧定喘胶囊治疗支气管哮喘的临床观察. 广西中医药. 1999,22(1):1–3
H38	梁镇忠, 罗丽琼, 梁丽卿. 平喘汤治疗支气管哮喘的临床疗效观察. 中国中医药咨讯. 2011,3(9):21–22
H39	李新. 益气固肺疏风法治疗支气管哮喘临床缓解期 30 例疗效观察. 北京中医药. 2011,30(4):290–291
H40	李小娟, 封继宏, 刘恩顺, 等. 补肺颗粒治疗哮喘缓解期疗效观察. 中国实验方剂学杂志. 2013,19(9):301–303
H41	李江文. 气管炎咳喘丸联合中药汤剂治疗支气管哮喘 64 例临床疗效观察. 当代医学. 2010,16(25):147
H42	黄益民, 丘革新, 陈秀霞, 等. 小青龙汤配合西药治疗哮证 (冷哮型) 的研究. 现代中西医结合杂志. 2006,15(9):1149–1150
H43	高雪, 曲敬来, 邱晨, 等. 小青龙汤改善冷哮型支气管哮喘气道重塑的临床研究. 中医药学报. 2006,34(6):20–22
H44	池少明. 老年哮喘的中医治疗. 中医临床研究. 2010,2(7):64–65
H45	陈云. 中西医结合治疗支气管哮喘临床观察. 中国社区医师· 医学专业. 2011,13(30):209
H46	陈晓勤, 张慧勇, 邵长荣, 等. 川芎平喘合剂治疗支气管哮喘 60 例. 江西中医药. 2009,40(3):41–42
H47	曹伟云. 参蛤散加味治疗缓解期老年支气管哮喘 45 例临床观察. 中医药导报. 2012,18(6):38–40
H48	蔡培勇, 谢苗苗. 二陈汤合三子养亲汤加味治疗痰湿蕴肺型喘证 50 例. 湖南中医杂志. 2013,29(2):35
H49	包成荣. 支气管哮喘中药治疗分析. 吉林医学. 2011,32(7):1304–1305
H50	柏晋梅, 杨爱枫. 清肺定喘胶囊治疗热哮型支气管哮喘临床观察. 山西中医. 2010,26(3):20–21
H51	张益康, 黄艳, 刘鑫, 等. 补肾活血汤治疗虚哮 30 例临床观察. 湖南中医杂志. 2008,24(2):23–24
H52	张文江, 苗青, 樊长征, 等. 辨证治疗支气管哮喘缓解期(肺脾气虚、肺肾两虚证)临床研究. 中国中医急症. 2012,21(1):14–16
H53	张伟江. 中医中药治疗慢性支气管哮喘的疗效分析. 求医问药. 2011,9(7):194

(*Continued*)

(Continued)

Study No.	References
H54	谢占武, 石福恒. 金匮肾气丸加味治疗支气管哮喘缓解期的临床疗效观察. 贵阳中医学院学报. 2014,36(2):66–68
H55	范欣生, 周志祥, 姜静, 等. 中药吸入治疗中轻度支气管哮喘的临床疗效及对血、痰中IL-8水平的影响. 中国医药学报. 2001,16(2):38–41
H56	杨嘉成. 补气定喘丸治疗支气管哮喘例60临床观察. 实用医学杂志. 1997,13(10):685
H57	杨继兵,严娴. 理肺补肾汤治疗支气管哮喘 50 例临床观察. 长春中医学院学报. 1998,14(70):5–6
H58	王志刚. 平喘汤治疗支气管哮喘临床观察. 河北中医. 2001,23(5):347
H59	王琦, 许德金, 许爱兰, 等. 上海丹参片治疗支气管哮喘的临床及实验研究. 实用中西医站台杂志. 1998,11(2):104–105
H60	乔世举, 于雪峰, 佟立君. 金水定喘汤治疗支气管哮喘 38 例临床观察. 实用中医内科杂志. 2002,16(2):91
H61	欧广升. 仙露喘哮康胶囊治疗支气管哮喘 5O 例临床观察. 湖南中医杂志. 1996,12(3):12–13
H62	刘辉. 金匮肾气丸辅助治疗非急性发作期哮喘 28 例. 杏林中医药. 2010,30(12):1059–1060
H63	黄忠远, 杨军平, 邱丽瑛. 解郁定喘汤治疗情志性支气管哮喘 22 例疗效观察. 山东医药. 2008,48(15):61
H64	黄大文, 李英姿, 俞军. 银杏苦内酯片治疗支气管哮喘临床观察. 长春中医学院学报. 2001,17(1):12,13
H65	Houssen M, Ragab E, Mesbah A, El-Samanoudy A, Othman AZ, Moustafa G, et al. Natural anti-inflammatory products and leukotriene inhibitors as complementary therapy for bronchial asthma. *Clin Biochem* 2010; 43(10–11):887–90.
H66	何晓春, 聂世来, 朱丽芳. 首乌喘息胶囊治疗哮喘的临床观察. 铁道医学. 1997;25(1):56
H67	耿志广, 郝风亮,毛学忠. 银杏叶片对缓解期哮喘患者气道高反应性及肺功能的影响. 临床荟萃. 1999,14(4):151–152
H68	方向明, 曹世宏. 平喘合剂治疗寒性哮喘的临床研究. 中国中医药科技. 2003,10(1):8–9
H69	单昌涛. 加味补中益气汤治疗支气管哮喘缓解期的临床观察. 河北中医. 2005,27(8):604

(Continued)

(Continued)

Study No.	References
H70	崔悦, 周旭生. 固本咳喘丸治疗激素依赖性支气管哮喘的临床观察. 中国中医药科技. 2001,8(3):189–190
H71	崔芳囡, 张燕萍. 麻红止哮汤治疗支气管哮喘慢性持续期的临床研究. 中国民间疗法. 2008,(12):25–26
H72	陈章生, 兰智慧, 丁雨红. 小青龙汤治疗上呼吸道感染诱发哮喘的临床观察. 实用中西医结合临床. 2011,11(3):22–23
H73	陈斯宁, 黄美杏, 梁爱武. 补肺汤治疗支气管哮喘及对免疫功能的影响. 陕西中医. 2009,30(8):939–940
H74	赵永辰, 韩玉娥, 高月平, 等. 中西医结合治疗过敏性哮喘疗效观察. 河北职工医学院学报. 2001,18(4):24–25
H75	Kim DH, Phillips JF, Lockey RF. Oral curcumin supplementation in patients with atopic asthma. *Allergy Rhinol* 2011;2(2):e51–3
H76	Nishizawa Y, Nishizawa Y, Yoshioka F. [Clinical effect of Chai-to-tang (Japanese name: Saiboku-to), a Chinese traditional herbal medicine, in patients with bronchial asthma and autonomic nerve dysfunction: A multicenter, randomised, double-blind, placebo-controlled study.]. Nihon Toyo Shinshin Igaku Kenkyu (*J Jap Assoc Oriental Psychosom Med*). 2004; 19:37–41
H77	邵长荣, 陈凤鸣, 唐忆星, 等. 川芎平喘合剂防治支气管哮喘的临床及实验研究. 中国中西医结合杂志. 1994,18(4):465–468
H78	Wen M, Wei C, Hu CH, Srivastava ZQ, Ko K, Xi J, Mu ST, et al. Efficacy and tolerability of antiasthma herbal medicine intervention in adult patients with moderate-severe allergic asthma. *J Allergy Clin Immunol* 2005,116(3):517–24
H79	钟亮环. 射麻止喘液治疗哮喘发作期的临床疗效观察及其对外周血IL-5, IL-8的影响[D]. 广州；广州中医药大学. 2005
H80	祝震天. 中西医结合治疗支气管哮喘6O例. 中国中医急症. 2010,19(4):660–661
H81	王梅, 赵家亮. 中药联合舒利迭治疗支气管哮喘非急性发作期的临床疗效观察. 湖北中医杂志. 2013,35(9):40
H82	周小华. 中西医结合治疗支气哮喘 60 例疗效观察. 世界中西医结合杂志. 2007,2(2):78
H83	钟勇. 养阴益肺汤联合舒利迭治疗支气管哮喘 68 例临床观察. 中国医药指南. 2010,8(13):133–134

(Continued)

Study No.	References
H84	郑海. 中药联合信必可都保治疗支气管哮喘 38 例临床观察. 国医论坛. 2011,26(2):29–30
H85	赵宗凯. 支气管哮喘采取中药灵芝补肺汤治疗的效果观察. 中国民康医学. 2013,25(15):71–72
H86	赵克明, 徐艳玲. 小柴胡汤加味合西药治疗支气管哮喘 43 例. 辽宁中医杂志. 2009,36(4):580–581
H87	赵杰, 金沈蓉, 王琰. 中西医结合治疗支气管哮喘 36 例临床观察. 四川中医. 2007,25(5):39–40
H88	赵建民. 三子养亲汤加味配合西药治疗支气管哮喘 68 例. 四川中医. 2009,27(5):89
H89	赵存杰. 中西医结合治疗老年支气管哮喘 48 例临床体会. 中国中医急症. 2009,18(11):1879
H90	章匀, 孙建. 疏风平哮汤配合布地奈德吸入治疗支气管哮喘疗效观察. 辽宁中医药大学大学学报. 2009,11(9):113–114
H91	张尊磊. 中西医结合治疗 40 例支气管哮喘患者的临床观察. 中国实用医药. 2012,7(7):144
H92	张招英, 赵明晶. 中西医结合治疗支气管哮喘的临床观察. 中医药学报. 2013,41(3):119–120
H93	张元元, 张燕萍, 王书臣, 等. 益肾活血平喘方药对哮喘患者病情控制水平和生命质量的影响. 现代中西医结合杂志. 2013,22(2):115,138
H94	张学燕. 射干麻黄汤加减治疗支气管哮喘 40 例. 河南中医. 2011,31(1):10–11
H95	张华平. 中西医结合治疗支气管哮喘疗效分析. 慢性病学杂志. 2010,12(10):1238–1239
H96	张鸿秋. 加味定喘汤治疗支气管哮喘72例疗效观察. 安徽医药. 2012,16(11):1666–1667
H97	张弘, 陈芳, 何薇, 等. 中西医结合治疗支气管哮喘缓解期临床观察. 浙江中医药大学学报. 2013,37(2):158–160
H98	张凤宇, 王超红, 李淑芳, 等. 麻杏甘石汤联合舒利迭治疗支气管哮喘(痰热壅肺证)临床观察. 中国中医急症.2011,20(3):364–365
H99	姚亮, 汤杰, 杨佩兰. 解痉祛风扶正法结合常规疗法治疗支气管哮喘慢性持续期临床观察. 上海中医药杂志. 2013,47(10):25–27
H100	杨志兰, 伍丽萍, 宦丽群. 综合治疗支气管哮喘慢性持续期和缓解期 32 例. 实用临床医学. 2009,10(9):28–29

(Continued)

(Continued)

Study No.	References
H101	谢帮军. 中西医结合治疗支气管哮喘疗效观察. 中国中医急症. 2005,14(9):835–836
H102	肖作清. 中西医结合治疗老年支气管哮喘疗效观察. 中国民康医学. 2011,23(8):964–965
H103	向建华, 毛良平, 韩鹏凯, 等. 沙美特罗替卡松联合金水宝胶囊治疗中度非急性发作期支气管哮喘 100 例临床观察.西部中医药. 2013,26(5):97–99
H104	武艳丽. 中西医结合治疗支气管哮喘 53 例临床观察. 中国医药指南. 2013,11(20):414–415
H105	武丹平. 中西医结合治疗支气管哮喘108例. 山西中医. 1997,13(1):15–16
H106	吴玉泓, 王清峰, 殷银霞, 等. 哮喘灵对支气管哮喘患者CD4+, CD8+ 及IgE的影响. 山东医药. 2008,48(4):85–86
H107	吴沛琴, 高洁. 中西医结合治疗哮喘 36 例. 山西中医. 2010,26(4):22
H108	温明春, 魏春华, 于农, 等. 中药灵芝补肺汤治疗支气管哮喘临床研究. 国际呼吸杂志. 2012,32(13):965–968
H109	魏小林. 三子养亲汤联合激素对哮喘患者尿白三烯E4水平的影响. 中医杂志. 2012,53(21):1831–1834
H110	魏春华, 温明春, 于农, 等. 柴朴颗粒联合常规疗法治疗难治性哮喘临床观察. 中国中西医结合杂志. 2011,31(1):33–36
H111	王雪慧, 刘建秋, 隋博文, 等. 温阳益气化痰平喘方治疗支气管哮喘慢性持续期 45 例临床观察. 中医药学报. 2013,41(1):102–103
H112	王文珍, 吴邦辉, 邢旭. 肺舒合剂治疗支气管哮喘急性发作期疗效观察. 中华中医药学刊. 2007,25(5):1076–1077
H113	王文慧, 赵洪波. 定喘汤对支气管哮喘患者肺功能及血清 IL-4 和ECT的影响. 河北中医. 2010,32(3):335–337
H114	王卫国. 自拟定哮平喘汤治疗老年支气管哮喘的临床疗效观察. 中国保健营养. 2010,(7): 87
H115	王宁群, 黄小波, 陈文强. 补益肺肾法对支气管哮喘疗效及患者生存质量的影响. 北京中医药. 2010,29(9):659–661
H116	王凯军. 中西医结合治疗寒性哮喘急性发作期肺功能观察 46 例. 中医研究. 2005,18(2):24–25
H117	王晶波, 彭先祝, 隋博文. 射干麻黄汤加味治疗难治性哮喘 33 例临床观察. 中医杂志. 2013,54(10):846–848
H118	王建平, 卢玫琳. 二龙麻杏汤联合西药治疗支气管哮喘42例. 中医研究. 2012,25(11):28–29

(Continued)

(Continued)

Study No.	References
H119	王辉, 邢慧芝, 宋丽红, 等. 清肺饮合百令胶囊为主治疗支气管哮喘的临床研究. 国际中医中药杂志. 2009,31(1):37–38
H120	田杰毅, 于素霞. 中西医结合治疗支气管哮喘 46 例. 上海中医药杂志. 2004,36(8):22–23
H121	陶荣菊. 补肾平喘汤联合西药治疗支气管哮喘 48 例临床观察. 云南中医中药杂志. 2011,32(11):44–46
H122	谭汉斌, 李刚. 中西医结合治疗支气管哮喘急性发作期 52 例临床观察. 中华医药杂志. 2004,4(3):254–255
H123	苏淑丹. 中西医结合治疗寒喘型支气管哮喘临床观察. 中国老年保健医学. 2012,10(5):15–16
H124	苏奎国, 张波, 姜良铎. 射干麻黄汤化裁联合舒利迭治疗哮喘 72 例疗效观察. 辽宁中医杂志. 2010,37(7):1273–1274
H125	石岫岩.加味止哮汤联合西药治疗支气管哮喘30例.南京中医药大学学报. 2012,28(6):589–590
H126	石静娟.小青龙汤加减配合西药治疗支气管哮喘40例.河南中医. 2009,29(12):1157–1158
H127	卿照前. 补中益气丸对老年支气管哮喘缓解期患者肺功能的影响. 湖南中医药大学学报. 2007,27(3):47–48
H128	亓庆胜, 李高云, 姜文, 等. 中药组方对哮喘患者的临床疗效观察. 医学理论与实践. 2007,20(9):1057–1058
H129	潘成琨. 中西医结合治疗老年性支气管哮喘疗效观察. 中国当代医药. 2011,18(27): 179–180
H130	聂媛媛. 中西医治疗支气管哮喘 52 例临床观察. 亚太传统医药. 2008,4(11):81–82
H131	倪健, 董竞成. 银杏内酯雾化吸入治疗支气管哮喘的临床研究. 中国中西医结合杂志. 2005,25(8): 696–699
H132	马谦, 黄庆田, 张国梁. 温肾防喘胶囊配合必可酮溶剂吸入治疗支气管哮喘的临床观察. 吉林中医药. 2007,27(8):23–24
H133	罗志泉. 补中益气汤联合舒利迭治疗支气管哮喘缓解期的临床疗效观察. 吉林医学. 2012,33(34):7497–7498
H134	鹿振辉, 张惠勇, 耿佩华, 等. 川芎平喘合剂联合西药治疗慢性持续期支气管哮喘临床研究. 2010,44(6):10–12

(Continued)

Study No.	References
H135	刘勤建. 中西医结合治疗老年支气管哮喘 45 例疗效分析. 中国中医药现代远程教育. 2009,(7): 22
H136	刘娟. 中西医结合治疗支气管哮喘临床观察. 辽宁中医药大学学报. 2009,11(5):138–139
H137	李智勇, 金鑫, 王静波. 中西医结合治疗支气管哮喘 32 例分析. 中医药学刊. 2004,22(3):523–524
H138	李影捷, 惠萍, 陈照南, 等. 温肾消喘膏方防治哮喘慢性持续期疗效观察. 新中医. 2013,45(4):37–39
H139	李晓霞. 中西医结合治疗支气管哮喘缓解期. 海峡药学. 2010,22(2):135–136
H140	李希, 严桂珍, 李大治. 中西医结合治疗支气管哮喘疗效观察. 药学进展. 2007,31(6): 280–282
H141	李文辉. 中西医结合治疗支气管哮喘的临床研究. 中国医药指南. 2010,8(3):104–105
H142	李平. 蛤蚧防喘丸治疗支气管哮喘临床研究. 中国中医急症. 2007,16(9):1055–1056
H143	李培伟. 平喘汤加减治疗支气管哮喘 32 例. 中国中医药现代远程教育. 2010,(10):11
H144	李莉. 中西医结合治疗支气管哮喘临床观察. 中国民族民间医药杂志. 2010,19(13): 152
H145	李景福. 辛夷, 苍耳子对支气管哮喘患者 Th1/Th2 比值及炎性递质的影响. 现代中西医结合杂志. 2012,21(10):1057–1058
H146	李海燕, 顾超, 汤杰, 等. 加味解痉祛风汤治疗支气管哮喘慢性持续期风哮证临床观察. 新中医. 2013,45(1): 26–29
H147	李风森, 白文梅. 祛风止痉散对哮喘风痰哮证患者肺功能, FeNo 的影响. 医学信息. 2012,25(8):60–61
H148	兰建阳. 五味平喘汤配合西药治疗支气管哮喘 65 例. 中国中医急症. 2011,20(12):2032–2033
H149	金丽萍, 徐霖伟. 补中益气汤联合舒利迭治疗支气管哮喘. 中国实验方剂学杂志. 2013,19(17):334–336
H150	金朝晖, 范伏元. 平哮定喘止咳汤治疗支气管哮喘临床观察. 中医临床研究. 2011,3(13):47–48

(Continued)

Study No.	References
H151	加米拉·沙依木, 热孜万古丽·阿帕尔, 廖洪利, 等. 舒肝解忧中药治疗支气管哮喘的临床分析. 右江医学. 2009,37(4):418–419
H152	黄焰, 刘峰林. 抗敏平喘汤联合药物吸入对支气管哮喘肺及免疫功能的影响. 内蒙古中医药. 2013,32(22): 22–23
H153	黄家聪. 加用小青龙汤合阳和汤治疗寒性支气管哮喘疗效观察. 广西中医药. 2012,35(6):30–31
H154	黄慧, 姚勇, 喻超英. 中药联合非特异性免疫药物治疗激素抵抗性哮喘 30 例疗效观察. 云南中医中药杂志. 2011,32(3):20–21
H155	黄慧, 姚勇, 喻超英. 非特异性免疫药物结合中药对激素抵抗性哮喘患者 Th1/Th2 细胞因子的影响. 中国现代药物应用. 2011,5(6):12–13
H156	黄苟根. 中西药联合治疗老年慢性哮喘的效果观察. 临床合理用药. 2013,6(10):52
H157	黄波, 李天禹, 秦建平, 等. 固本平喘汤治疗支气管哮喘慢性持续期 48 例. 中国实验方剂学杂志. 2013,19(20):277–280
H158	胡建荣. 中西医结合治疗慢性持续期支气管哮喘 53 例. 基层医学论坛. 2012,16(10): 1315–1316
H159	何乐. 孟鲁司特钠联合蛤蚧定喘胶囊治疗支气管哮喘疗效分析. 中国误诊学杂志. 2008,8(29):7089–7090
H160	郭玉莉. 喘苏荨颗粒治疗支气管哮喘 49 例疗效观察. 上海中医药杂志. 2013,47(1):39–40
H161	冯春林. 中西药联合治疗支气管哮喘临床观察. 中医药学刊. 2005,23(8):1532
H162	房体静, 冉宝兴, 严宏彬. 中西医结合治疗支气管哮喘的效果及对免疫功能的影响. 中医药导报. 19(9):2013,19(9):48–50
H163	范海军. 补肺汤治疗支气管哮喘慢性持续期效果观察. 光明中医. 2012,27(12):2461–2462
H164	范德斌, 秦雪屏, 白红华, 等. 咳喘停袋泡颗粒治疗热哮型支气管哮喘 43 例临床研究. 云南中医中药杂志. 2010,31(8):14–15
H165	段建萍. 中西医结合治疗支气管哮喘 46 例疗效观察. 云南中医中药杂志. 2005,26(2):6–7
H166	董滟, 穆晓翌, 王钢. 哮平 I 号方治疗支气管哮喘的临床研究. 四川中医. 2012,30(12):61–64

(Continued)

(Continued)

Study No.	References
H167	崔红生, 徐光勤, 任传云, 等. 激素依赖型哮喘撤减激素过程中的证候学变化及三步序贯法临床疗效观察. 中医杂志. 2008,49(10):886–889
H168	崔红生, 崔巍, 温志浩, 等. 三步序贯法对激素依赖型哮喘患者 T 辅助细胞亚群的影响. 中国中西医结合杂志. 2006,26(12):1074–1077
H169	楚洪生. 综合疗法在支气管哮喘治疗中的临床应用. 中国保健营养·临床医学学刊. 2010,19(7): 140–141
H170	陈雪梅. 麻杏定喘汤治疗支气管哮喘临床效果研究. 亚太传统医药. 2013,9(7):142–143
H171	陈旭明, 宁观林, 彭观娣. 平喘汤联合西药治疗支气管哮喘的疗效观察. 临床医学工程. 2010,17(4):101–102
H172	陈维力. 中西医结合治疗支气管哮喘 63 例疗效观察. 中华实用医学. 2004,6(10):39–40
H173	陈平保. 平喘汤结合舒利迭治疗支气管哮喘 50 例疗效观察. 中医临床研究. 2012,4(11):64–65
H174	陈科伶, 董滟, 陶陶. 调肝理肺法辅助治疗肝郁型哮喘的临床研究. 四川中医. 2013,31(4):65–67
H175	曹雅静. 氨茶碱伍用知母对支气管哮喘患者血清一氧化氮含量的影响. 实用心脑肺血管病杂志. 2006, 14(3): 210
H176	周礼双. 中药汤剂加减联合西医治疗慢性支气管哮喘对照研究. 实用中医内科杂志. 2012,26(11):14–15
H177	钟敏, 陈生. 柴朴颗粒联合西医治疗难治性哮喘应用分析. 吉林医学. 2012,33(6):1191–1192
H178	张玉霞, 朱运波, 宫玉凤. 三种治疗老年过敏性哮喘病方剂对比研究. 中国药物经济学. 2013(4):275–277
H179	张锐. 平喘汤配合西药治疗支气管哮喘 56 例. 辽宁中医药大学学报. 2009,11(4):120–121
H180	姚青平. 30 例中西医结合治疗支气管哮喘临床观察. 求医问药. 2012,10(1):185
H181	徐波. 应用射干麻黄汤治疗支气管哮喘 30 例的临床效果观察. 求医问药. 2013,11(6):175–176
H182	夏露华. 止哮救肺汤联合布地奈德气雾剂治疗哮喘疗效观察. 实用中医内科杂志. 2012,26(7):28–29

(Continued)

(Continued)

Study No.	References
H183	汪旭华, 钟小兵, 许强. 中医治疗支气管哮喘的临床疗效观察. 求医问药. 2013,11(6):167
H184	唐百冬, 屈娅婷. 定喘汤化裁方配合西药治疗治疗支气管哮喘(热哮) 35 例临床观察. 中国医药指南. 2008,24(6):188–189
H185	宿英豪, 苏奎国, 马蕴蕾, 等. 补益肺肾、化饮通络法治疗支气管哮喘缓解期的临床效果. 中国中医基础医学杂志. 2013,19(11):1323–1325
H186	林茂华, 杨清儒, 邓彪, 等. 右归饮汤剂对难治性哮喘患者血浆皮质醇及免疫球蛋白水平的影响. 临床和实验医学杂志. 2007,6(2):129–130
H187	廖泽安. 小青龙汤在治疗呼吸内科疾病中的应用. 求医问药. 2013,11(8):166–167
H188	李强, 钟连英, 胡燕明, 等. 补肾止喘冲剂对难治性哮喘皮质醇和哮喘发作的作用. 实用医学杂志. 2006,22(21):2548–2550
H189	李岚生. 止咳平喘中药联合西药治疗支气管哮喘随机平行对照研究. 实用中医内科杂志. 2013,27(9):51–54
H190	黄启辉, 江山平, 陈广穗, 等. 雷公藤甲素对激素抵抗型哮喘患者血清 Th2 细胞因子水平和肺功能的影响. 中国中医药科技. 2003,10(2):72–73
H191	洪根华. 中西医结合治疗慢性持续期老年支气管哮喘的疗效分析. 求医问药. 2013,11(4):335
H192	韩玲. 中西医结合治疗支气管哮喘 69 例. 中国中医药现代远程教育. 2013,11(21):45
H193	沈炳煌, 沈良秀, 范小山. 中西医结合治疗支气管哮喘缓解期临床观察. 福建医药杂志. 2007,29(4):123–124
H194	申燕华. 中西医结合治疗寒喘型支气管哮喘临床效果观察. 求医问药. 2013,11(2):324–325
H195	邹萍. 自拟定喘汤治疗老年支气管哮喘发作 90 例临床疗效分析. 中国中医基础医学杂志. 2008,14(10):784
H196	周庆伟. 中西医结合治疗重症哮喘 30 例. 河南中医学院学报. 2005,20(4):51–52
H197	曾广田. 中西医结合治疗支气管哮喘 3O 例疗效观察. 河南中医. 2004,24(5):47–48
H198	余月芳, 吴国水. 定喘汤治疗热哮疗效观察. 浙江中西医结合杂志. 2007,17(1):33–34
H199	余国英, 李敬会, 李华云. 地龙汤治疗老年支气管哮喘临床体会. 中国中医急症. 2006,15(9):1037–1038

(Continued)

Study No.	References
H200	杨周瑞. 补肾止喘汤治疗支气管哮喘的临床研究. 辽宁中医药大学学报. 2007,9(2):84–85
H201	吴孝田. 六味地黄丸加味治疗激素依赖性哮喘临床观察. 辽宁中医学院学报. 2005,7(6):587
H202	吴淑红. 中西医结合治疗支气管哮喘 58 例临床观察. 浙江中西医结合杂志. 2005,15(7):428–429
H203	吴淑红. 中西医结合治疗支气管哮喘疗效观察. 浙江中西医结合杂志. 2000,10(11):667–668
H204	王震. 参蛤定喘胶囊的制备及临床疗效观察. 湖北中医杂志. 2013,35(11):76–77
H205	王真, 杨琚超, 宫晓燕, 等. 清肺平喘补肾颗粒治疗 144 例哮喘轻度持续患者疗效观察. 中华中医药杂志. 2013,28(2):351–353
H206	王丽红. 中西医结合治疗赠治性哮喘的临床研究. 卫生职业教育. 2006,24(16):146–147
H207	王华忠. 中西医结合治疗支气管哮喘 68 例临床观察. 湖南中医药学报. 2000,6(10):25
H208	邱新英, 叶敏和. 中西医结合治疗老年人轻中度慢性持续期哮喘临床效果分析. 中国基层医药. 2013,20(16):2523–2525
H209	乔世举, 李可畏, 伊艳杰. 中西医结合治疗支气管哮喘临床观察. 辽宁中医杂志. 2002,29(6):352
H210	钱锐. 中西医结合治疗支气管哮喘 36 例临床观察. 中国中医药科技. 2005,12(2):114–115
H211	欧晓芳. 中西医结合治疗支气管哮喘 50 例. 河南中医. 2007,27(11):60–61
H212	罗庆东, 于湘春, 李素兰. 自拟涤痰定喘汤治疗支气管哮喘急性发作 40 例疗效观察. 黑龙江中医药. 2004,4:20–21
H213	刘永平. 基本方加减配合西药治疗痰热型支气管哮喘疗效观察. 陕西中医. 2011,32(12):1626–1627
H214	刘淮, 李川申, 邹芬芳. 黄喘平超大剂量雾化吸入治疗支气管哮喘疗效观察. 湖北中医杂志. 2005,27(12):26
H215	刘丹. 小青龙汤治疗寒性支气管哮喘 30 例临床观察. 中国医学研究与临床. 2006,4(4):67–68
H216	刘春平. 中西医结合治疗支气管哮喘的疗效观察. 中国中医药咨讯. 2010,2(32):208,215

(Continued)

(Continued)

Study No.	References
H217	林晓英, 严子兴. 自拟麻龙平喘汤治疗过敏性哮喘 40 例. 海峡药学. 2008,20(8):130–131
H218	李战炜. 72 例支气管哮喘的中西医结合治疗结果分析. 2012,10(21):240–241
H219	李雪珍, 陈治林. 中西医结合治疗支气管哮喘 69 例临床观察. 现代医药卫生, 2005,21(12):1562–1563
H220	李川申, 郭际, 钱育梅. 黄喘平雾化剂经加压超声雾化吸入治疗支气管哮喘的临床观察. 中国全科医学杂志. 1999,2(4):296–298
H221	金晓滢, 楼建国, 詹小萍, 等. 气管舒合剂治疗支气管哮喘的临床观察. 中国中药杂志. 2007,3(21)79–81
H222	姜静, 范欣生, 尚宁, 等. 复方辛夷口服液在支气管哮喘治疗中的应用. 南京中医药大学学报, 2002,28(6):333–334
H223	季红燕, 王胜, 朱春冬, 等. 麻贝汤治疗难治性哮喘 9 例. 山东中医杂志. 2011,30(9):628–629
H224	黄笑娟, 黄纪文, 冯艳翠. 中西医结合治疗老年慢性持续期哮喘 158 例临床观察. 中医药指南. 2012,10(17):285–286
H225	黄湘霞. 平喘抗敏汤治疗过敏性哮喘 42 例.四川中医. 2002,20(7):44
H226	黄开珍, 王朝晖, 黄美杏, 等. 加味小青龙汤联合常规西药治疗支气管哮喘急性发作期32例. 广西医科大学学报. 2008,25(5):788–789
H227	胡为营. 自拟喘舒汤治疗缓解期难治性支气管哮喘 60 例临床观察. 河北中医. 2005,27(7):512
H228	杭东辉, 中西医结合治疗支气管哮喘 40 例临床观察. 江苏中医药. 2003,24(10):26
H229	高轶峰, 林秀菊, 万丹. 中西药联合佐治 120 例支气管哮喘临川研究. 中国医药导刊. 2011,13(3):460–461
H230	邓盛英. 中西医联合治疗重度支气管哮喘的临床疗效观察. 医学理论与实践. 2013,26(22):2990–2991
H231	崔红生, 武维屏, 任传云, 等. 加减乌梅丸治疗激素依赖型哮喘 20 例临床疗效观察.中国中医基础医学杂志. 2004,10(8):49–50
H232	程荣朵, 赵木昆, 冉洪强. 射干麻黄汤配合西药治疗支气管哮喘 46 例. 陕西中医. 2005,26(4):294–295
H233	程德华, 汪晖云. 中西医结合治疗支气管哮喘 160 例. 陕西中医. 1999,20(3):104–105

(Continued)

(Continued)

Study No.	References
H234	陈晓明. 舒肝解忧汤剂治疗支气管哮喘 90 例临床分析. 亚太传统医药. 2012,8(4):155–156
H235	陈小英. 34 例支气管哮喘的临床分析. 医学信息. 2011,24(7):4176–4177
H236	刘丽, 李宏伟. 中西医结合治疗支气管哮喘 46 例. 黑龙江中医药. 2001,(3): 35
H237	Song KG, Shen XY, Wang HH, Yang Z, Luo JC, Cao XF, *et al*. Randomised controlled study on qingfei pingchuan bushen keli for treatment of chronic duration of asthma. Respirology Conference: 16th Congress of the Asian Pacific Society of Respirology Shanghai China 3–6 November 2011. 2011; 16(Suppl 2):202–3
H238	Tang B, Shi K, Li X, Wang H, Fang H, Xiong B, Wu Y.Effect of "yang-warming and kidney essence-replenishing" herbal paste on cold-related asthma exacerbation. *J Trad Chine Med* 2014; 33(4):468–72
H239	Thomas M, Sheran J, Smith N, Fonseca S, Lee AJ. AKL1, a botanical mixture for the treatment of asthma: a randomised, double-blind, placebo-controlled, cross-over study. *BMC Pulm Med* 2007; 7:4
H240	Wang G, Zhang HP, Jia CE, Liang R, Cheng Y. Traditional chinese medicine for treatment of acute asthma: A randomised, double-blind, placebo-controlled trial. *Respirology* 2012;17:14
H241	Zha Q, Lin S, Zhang C, Chang C, Xue H, Lu C. Xiaoqinglong granules as add-on therapy for asthma: latent class analysis of symptom predictors of response. *Evid Based Complement Alternat Med* 2013;2013:759476
H242	杨吉. 通腑活血法联合舒利迭治疗支气管哮喘的临床研究[D]. 南京:南京中医药大学. 2011
H243	吴琼. 加味三子养亲汤治疗支气管哮喘慢性持续期(痰阻气奎证)临床研究[D]. 武汉: 湖北中医药大学. 2010
H244	陈晨. 探讨病证结合治疗支气管哮喘的临床疗效[D]. 南京: 南京中医药大学. 2012
H245	王艳玲. 防哮饮对哮喘慢性持续期患者的临床疗效研究[D]. 南宁: 广西中医学院. 2011
H246	田乃妲, 张超. 敏喘平胶囊治疗支气管哮喘的临床研究. 天津中医. 1994,11(6):38–39
H247	孙增涛张, 唐饴环, 高凤琴, 张虹,. 杏贝冲剂治疗支气管哮喘临床疗效分析. 哮喘与肺部疾病. 1996;(3):5–8

(Continued)

(Continued)

Study No.	References
H248	童瑾 王. 平喘汤与舒利迭对支气管哮喘缓解期疗效比较的研究. 激光杂志. 2011;32(3):82–3
H249	刘世昌. 自拟止哮平喘汤治疗支气管哮喘 40 例. 国医论坛. 2006;21(2):26
H250	陈勇平 刘. 鲜竹沥雾化吸入治疗哮喘的临床观察. 药学实践杂志. 2003;21(1):5
H251	王济梅. 补气活血方治疗支气管哮喘 32 例疗效观察. 中医药研究. 1999;;15(6):20–1
H252	刘茵. 补肺汤加减治疗哮证缓解期临床研究. 中医临床研究. 2011;3(6):24–5
H253	赵国萍. 中西医结合治疗老年哮喘的疗效观察. 当代医学. 2010;16(34):142–3
H254	曾红梅. 平喘汤佐治老年支气管哮喘 80 例. 陕西中医. 2012;33(7):829
H255	李琼芳. 补肺汤治疗支气管哮喘慢性持续期的临床疗效. 中外医学研究. 2013;11(28):44–5
H256	忻璐洁. 中西医结合治疗支气管哮喘慢性持续期疗效观察. 浙江中西医结合杂志. 2012;22(12):961–3
H257	吴孝田. 六味地黄丸合参蛤散为主治疗激素依赖性哮喘 42 例-附单用西药治疗 39 例对照. 浙江中医杂志. 2005;40(10):427
H258	莎玫武. 麻射蝉葶汤治疗支气管哮喘临床观察. 内蒙古中医药. 2005;24(6):1
H259	陈刚庆. 老年支气管哮喘慢性持续期的治疗分析. 中国社区医师·医学专业. 2012;14(14):70
H260	孙碧雄张洪熹汪素蟾陈爱珍. 张伯臾治哮喘方疗效观察. 中西医结合杂志. 1990;(01):42–3
H261	朱慧志 季, 张念志,王胜,陈炜,杨程,. 阳和平喘颗粒对支气管哮喘慢性持续期寒哮证气道炎症的影响. 中医药临床杂志. 2010;(4):310–2
H262	周明萍 吕. 布地奈德联合金水宝胶囊治疗支气管哮喘的疗效观察. 临床军医杂志. 2012;40(4):954–5
H263	陈永莉 黄, 徐新华,. 定哮平喘液治疗支气管哮喘的临床效果研究. 中医临床研究. 2013;5(10):80,2
H264	牛秀清 牛. 中西医结合治疗支气管哮喘的临床观察. 中国实用医药. 2012;7(30):177–8
H265	郑玉琼 尹, 张爱平,贾波,. 平喘合剂治疗支气管哮喘热哮证的临床观察. 四川中医. 2006;24(10):58–9

(Continued)

(*Continued*)

Study No.	References
H266	张志文 马, 孙建君,陈晓霞,. 自拟补肺定喘汤对支气管哮喘缓解期的疗效观察. 宁夏医科大学学报. 2009;31(2):258–9
H267	张彦峰. 补中益气汤加减治疗支气管哮喘 21 例疗效观察. 长春中医药大学学报. 2008;24(2):191
H268	张家骝 姚, 张静珊,. 蝉地二陈汤加吸入疗法治疗轻中度哮喘 42 例疗效观察. 云南中医中药杂志. 2005;26(2):32–3
H269	余传星 王, 严桂珍,. 藿香正气散治疗寒哮 38 例. 新中医. 1999;31(1):31–2
H270	殷银霞. 桂枝加厚朴杏子汤治疗支气管哮喘 46 例临床观察. 甘肃中医学院学报. 2003;20(3):36–7
H271	闫德志. 中西医结合治疗支气管哮喘 81 例. 中国中医药现代远程教育. 2012;10(24):35–6
H272	许得盛 王, 陈伟华,. 桂龙咳喘宁胶囊治疗激素依赖性哮喘疗效观察. 浙江中西医结合杂志. 2002;12(5):277–8
H273	徐立然王, 金路,郑志攀,. 清养化痰方治疗 41 例支气管哮喘慢性持续期(肺肾阴虚, 痰热内蕴证)患者的临床观察. 辽宁中医杂志. 2011;38(5):908–10
H274	徐立然 王, 金路,郑志攀,. 温养化痰方治疗 60 例支气管哮喘慢性持续期患者的临床观察. 中华中医药杂志. 2011;26(4):868–9
H275	王洋. 自拟止咳平喘汤联合西药治疗支气管哮喘持续期 55 例. 实用中医内科杂志. 2012;26(10):21,3
H276	王立君. 过敏煎加味方治疗过敏性支气管哮喘 20 例. 江西中医药. 2008;39(11):21–4
H277	王宏长 吴, 唐斌擎,方泓,李晓琦,. 温阳补肾填精膏方治疗支气管哮喘的临床观察. 上海中医药杂志. 2008;42(11):28–9
H278	田爱荣. 加味小青龙汤治疗慢性哮喘 46 例临床观察. 中原医刊. 2003;30(18):11–2
H279	罗凤鸣 何, 杜建,. 加味肾气丸对支气管哮喘气道炎症抑制作用的临床研究. 中国中医药信息杂志. 2001;8(8):20–1
H280	李经杭. 定喘汤加减治疗支气管哮喘 78 例. 长春中医药大学学报. 2010;26(2):222
H281	杜丽娟 李. 定喘汤加味对支气管哮喘患者肺功能影响的研究. 新疆中医药. 2009;(5):6–7

(*Continued*)

(Continued)

Study No.	References
H282	单要军 薛, 李连,. 咳喘合剂治疗哮喘 108 例. 中医药学刊. 2004;22(11):2148
H283	崔静. 自拟红景五子定喘汤治疗支气管哮喘 60 例. 四川中医. 2012;30(11):98–9
H284	曹祥. 四子定喘汤治疗难治性哮喘 58 例. 中医药临床杂志. 2012;24(9):842
H285	周淳. 中西医结合治疗支气管哮喘 60 例临床分析. 现代中西医结合杂志. 2000;(02):65–6
H286	张慧. 调气平喘汤治疗支气管哮喘 100 例. 中国中医药现代远程教育. 2013;(20):134–5
H287	云少敏. 麻杏薏甘汤加味治疗支气管哮喘. 河南中医. 1999;(04):13
H288	王雨雁刘姝贾维刚. 自拟克喘煎治疗支气管哮喘 36 例. 中医药信息. 1999;(01):31
H289	陈兰云陈金广. 寒哮乐口服液治疗寒哮 105 例疗效分析. 临床医学. 1997;(07):19
H290	舒全政. 中医治疗哮喘的临床疗效观察. 大众健康：理论版. 2012;(10):120
H291	张诚. 五味咳喘停辨证治疗慢性哮喘 50 例. 中国中医药现代远程教育. 2010;(16):34–5
H292	张惠勇 梁, 田文英,吴银根,. 健脾温肾法膏方治疗支气管哮喘 65 例. 新中医. 1996;28(10):42–3
H293	赵蓓 潘. "祛风止痉化痰方"治疗支气管哮喘风痰哮证 40 例. 江苏中医药. 2010;42(10):51
H294	张清奇. 化瘀定喘汤治疗顽固性哮喘 46 例临床观察. 内蒙古中医药. 2006;25(4):14–5
H295	张芬兰 姜, 魏婷,. 疏肝理肺法治疗支气管哮喘 30 例临床观察. 长春中医学院学报. 2002;18(3):13–4
H296	张波. 参蛤散合射干麻黄汤加减治疗哮喘 64 例. 陕西中医. 2011;32(4):397–8
H297	袁天平. 化痰平喘汤治疗支气管哮喘 30 例临床观察. 中国中医药咨讯. 2011;3(2):81
H298	严忠. 麻龙汤治疗支气管哮喘 68 例疗效观察. 浙江中医学院学报. 1995;19(6):15
H299	吴健卫 赵, 曾灵芝,薛汉荣,洪广祥,. 温阳益气护卫汤预防哮喘发作的临床研究. 中华中医药杂志. 2005;20(7):434–6

(Continued)

(Continued)

Study No.	References
H300	王立茹. 三子养亲汤治疗支气管哮喘 120 例. 四川中医. 2012;30(4):84
H301	谭秀芳. 中西药综合治疗缓解期支气管哮喘效果评价. 医学创新研究. 2008;5(12):101–2
H302	孙增涛 唐, 张素仙,高凤琴,. 杏贝定喘汤治疗支气管哮喘 56 例疗效分析. 天津中医. 1996;13(2):29–30
H303	苏彩凤 崔. 平肝哮喘汤治疗支气管哮喘 60 例. 陕西中医. 2005;26(12):1271
H304	宋歌. 参芪定喘汤治疗支气管哮喘 32 例. 中国中医急症. 2007;16(8):999
H305	时以营. 止哮汤治疗支气管哮喘 36 例. 湖南中医杂志. 2007;23(2):70,6
H306	罗国蓉. 麻杏石甘汤治疗支气管哮喘 35 例临床体会. 按摩与康复医学. 2012;3(29):184–5
H307	路聚更 姜. 中药治疗激素依赖型支气管哮喘 65 例临床观察. 河北中医. 2005;27(5):343–4
H308	刘勇 蒋. 射干麻黄汤加味结合西药治疗支气管哮喘疗效观察. 内蒙古中医药. 2013;32(18):3
H309	刘建秋 聂, 赵丽芬,韩冰,. 克喘素冲剂治疗支气管哮喘 31 例临床观察. 中医药信息. 1999;16(5):20
H310	林欣江 臧. 中西医结合治疗支气管哮喘 64 例. 中国现代药物应用. 2009;3(2):90
H311	李寿庆. 阳和汤辨治哮喘夏季发作的体会——附 40 例临床观察. 内蒙古中医药. 2007;26(3):15
H312	黎同明 刘, 孙志佳,梁直英,. 定喘汤治疗热哮型哮喘 31 例. 陕西中医. 2005;26(4):293–4
H313	黄振达. 小青龙汤加味治疗老年支气管哮喘临床观察. 河北中医. 2004;26(4):249
H314	黄建平. 通宣理肺丸与酮替芬联用治疗支气管哮喘 27 例. 中国中西医结合急救杂志. 2013;20(4):251
H315	胡学芳 郎, 喻少峰,王欢,周思举,龚宣碧,. 经方治疗哮证发作期 30 例临床观察. 四川中医. 2008;26(8):76–7
H316	崔娣. "平喘汤"配合治疗哮喘 36 例. 江苏中医药. 2008;40(11):68
H317	陈维初. 调肝理肺汤治疗支气管哮喘 38 例疗效观察. 湖南中医杂志. 1997;13(5):12

(Continued)

(Continued)

Study No.	References
H318	陈成 唐, 曲建强,陈应贤,. 哮喘宁合剂的制备与临床疗效观察. 中药材. 1994;17(6):48–9
H319	曹方会. 祛风解痉法治疗支气管哮喘 100 例. 实用中医药杂志. 2010;(4):230–1
H320	蔡娟 武, 韩月香,. 麻黄鱼腥草汤治疗支气管哮喘缓解期 60 例临床观察. 山西中医学院学报. 2003; 4(3):12
H321	张金磊傅宏北黄爱贞王长印刘永丰尹文雄. 中药治疗激素依赖型哮喘 121 例. 中医杂志. 2000;(11):696
H322	曾庆华. 14 例"支气管哮喘"中医药治疗的临床分析. 江西医学院学报. 1959;(02):17–9
H323	余军，段天英. 参蛤三七散治疗顽固性支气管哮喘. 山西中医. 1994;(05):19–20
H324	严颖徐志瑛. 徐志瑛治疗支气管哮喘经验. 浙江中医药大学学报. 2013;(05):522–3+6
H325	李忠敏. 46 例自拟中药汤治疗顽固性哮喘临床观察. 中国实用医药. 2007;(16):105
H326	冀文鹏程书银. 辨证治疗哮喘 45 例临床观察. 中原医刊. 1991;(04):32–3
H327	李竹英 张, 关永杰,李世哲,吴树亮,. 定喘汤加减治疗支气管哮喘 60 例临床观察. 中医药学报. 1996; (6):15
H328	李慧. 温胆汤加减治疗支气管哮喘 56 例. 河北中医. 2002;24(5):365
H329	姜越 江. 江柏华教授治疗支气管哮喘经验. 黑龙江中医药. 2012;41(5):30–1
H330	于雪峰. 郭振武中药干预支气管哮喘缓解期经验探析. 辽宁中医杂志. 2009;(5):676–7
H331	常义. 中药治疗支气管哮喘 96 例临床观察. 中国社区医师·医学专业. 2012;14(18):221
H332	成怡楠. 平哮颗粒治疗支气管哮喘(风痰阻肺证)的临床研究. 2012
H333	Park CS, Kim TB, Lee JY, Park JY, Lee YC, Jeong SS *et al*. Effects of add-on therapy with NDC-052, an extract from Magnoliae Flos, in adult asthmatic patients receiving inhaled corticosteroids. *Korean J Intern Med* 2012;27(1):84–90

6

Pharmacological Actions of the Frequently Used Herbs

OVERVIEW

Herbs have pharmacological actions that may mediate the pathological processes in asthma, namely inflammation and airways hyperresponsiveness. The ten most frequently used herbs in the randomised clinical trials (see Chapter 5) were reviewed to examine their pharmacological actions. The common herbs in the clinical trials were *ma huang* 麻黄, *gan cao* 甘草, *xing ren* 杏仁, *ban xia* 半夏, *di long* 地龙, *zi su zi* 紫苏子, *huang qin* 黄芩, *wu wei zi* 五味子, *xi xin* 细辛, and *huang qi* 黄芪. Findings from experimental research highlight their treatment potential and provide some possible explanations for their clinical effects. Their actions and phytochemical constituents are summarised in relation to their effects on inflammation.

Introduction

Chinese herbs and medicinal formulae exert their actions through active constituent compounds. Experimental evidence helps to explain the possible mechanisms underlying the effects of the herbs on asthma. Experimental (*in vivo* and *in vitro*) evidence for a selection of the most frequently used herbs was reviewed in detail to determine how their biochemical properties contribute to their reported clinical benefits in people with asthma.

Experimental Studies on ma huang 麻黄

Ephedrine and pseudo-ephedrine are the two main compounds in *ma huang* 麻黄 (*Ephedra sinica* Stapf). Ephedrine is an adrenoceptor agonist that also increases norepinephrine release. *Ma huang* can stimulate the central nervous system and can function as a decongestant and bronchodilator. However, it has some reported side effects and should not be used long-term.[1] In relation to inflammation, the formula, *Ma huang tang* 麻黄汤, reduced airways resistance and reduced the number of eosinophils and interleukin (IL)-4 and IL-17 in an asthma mouse model.[2] The results showed that *Ma huang tang* 麻黄汤 can modulate T helper cell (Th1/Th2) cytokines and reduce the progress of allergic asthma.[2]

Experimental Studies on gan cao 甘草

Gan cao 甘草 (*Glycyrrhiza uralensis* Fisch., *Glycyrrhiza inflata* Bat., *Glycyrrhiza glabra* L.) contains many biologically active constituents known to have anti-inflammatory, antiviral, and antimicrobial actions.[3] In an asthma mouse model, *gan cao*'s constituent compound, glycyrrhizinic acid, reduced airway resistance and suppressed the generation of a Th2-type immune response, therefore reducing inflammation in the lungs.[4] *Gan cao* also possesses anti-tussive effects. An extract, liquiritin apioside, reduced cough in guinea pigs by acting on peripheral receptors in the airway and central receptors in the serotonergic system.[5]

Experimental Studies on xing ren 杏仁

Xing ren 杏仁 (*Prunus armeniaca* L.) contains several active compounds, such as the glycoside amygdalin, amygdalase, and arachidic acid. Anti-inflammation and anti-oxidation are commonly reported effects of *xing ren*. Several studies have documented *xing ren*'s effects in anti-cancer models, which may have implications for other types of inflammation including those seen in asthma.[6] *Xing ren* compounds, amygdalin and oleic acid, also have anti-oxidant effects.

Oleic acid reduced cellular oxidation and reactive oxygen species (ROS) by down-regulation of glutathione peroxidase.[7]

Experimental Studies on ban xia 半夏

Ban xia 半夏 (*Pinellia ternata* (Thunb.) Breit.) contains several groups of compounds including triterpenes, volatile oils, and phytosteroles.[8] One form of phytosteroles, β-sitosterol, was shown to reduce lipid peroxidation in rats by increasing anti-oxidant enzymes, catalase, superoxide dismutase, and glutathione peroxidase, in turn reducing oxidative stress.[9] β-sitosterol also reduced eosinophils, intracellular ROS, and cytokines IL-4 and IL-5 in an asthmatic mouse model.[10]

Experimental Studies on di long 地龙

Di long 地龙 (*Pheretima aspergillum* Perrier) is primarily composed of amino acids, xanthenes, and lipids.[11] *Di long* fractions reduced histamine-induced contraction of tracheal rings and protected guinea pigs from asthma induced by histamine and acetylcholine chloride, and also reduced cough frequency in mice.[12] An earthworm species similar to *di long*, *Lampito mauritii*, showed a reduction in inflammation and restoration of normal histamine levels that were induced by inflammation in a rat model.[13] Although the inflammatory model tested was not related to asthma, results showed positive anti-inflammatory effects and highlight the potential of *di long*. Xanthines are commonly used for asthma and xanthine drugs have been developed from other plants, such as cromoglycate.[14] Although there are currently no experimental studies evaluating xanthines from *di long*, these compounds plausibly account for some of its therapeutic effects in asthma.

Experimental Studies on zi su zi 紫苏子

Zi su zi 紫苏子 (*Perilla frutescens* L., *Perilla crispa* (Thunb.) Hand.-Mazz.) has several constituent compounds, including flavonoids (shisonin and vicenin), volatile oils, and amino acids.[11] In asthma experimental models, it reduced allergic responses by increasing IL-10 and reducing the Th2 immune response.[15] The seed oil has also shown significant anti-asthmatic effects. In sensitised guinea pigs, *zi su zi* oil dose-dependently reduced inflammatory cells, such as leukocytes and eosinophils, and reduced leukotriene release from the lungs.[16] *Zi su zi* oil given to people with asthma for four weeks also reduced leukotrines and reduced asthmatic impact by improving respiratory function and lipometabolism.[17] In another study, *zi su zi* was injected into the acupuncture point ST36 *Zusanli* 足三里 in mice.[18] The results showed that it reduced inflammatory cells in the lung and bronchoalveolar lavage fluid (BALF), and also reduced immunoglobulin E (IgE) and Th2 cytokines in BALF and serum, leading to an overall reduction in pathological changes in lung tissue.[18] Taken together, these results indicate that *zi su zi* has anti-asthmatic inflammatory and immune-regulatory effects by reducing eosinophilic inflammation and Th2 cytokines.

Experimental Studies on huang qin 黄芩

Huang qin 黄芩 (*Scutellaria baicalensis* Georgi) contains flavonoids (baicalin, wogonin, and norwogonin), glycosides (baicalin), volatile oils, phytosteroles, and amino acid.[8,11] The glycoside baicalin is a bioactive compound and reportedly has anti-inflammatory, anti-oxidant and anti-bacterial properties.[19,20] In cigarette-smoke exposed inflammatory models (*in vivo* and *in vitro*), baicalin had a significant anti-inflammatory effect by reducing pro-inflammatory mediators.[20] Wogonin has also shown anti-inflammatory effects by inducing eosinophil apoptosis and reducing allergic airway inflammation in mice.[21] Wogonin reduced eosinophils, mucus production, as well as inhibited airway hyperresponsiveness.[21] It was suggested that wogonin has therapeutic potential for treating allergic inflammation. In another study, *huang qin* reduced the expression of oxidants (inducible nitric oxide synthase, iNOS) and lessened inflammatory mediator synthesis (IL-1, IL-2, IL-6, IL-12, tumour necrosis factor -α). The authors showed that *huang qin* had significant anti-inflammatory effects.[22]

Experimental Studies on wu wei zi 五味子

Bioactive constituents of *wu wei zi* 五味子 (*Schisandra chinensis* (Turcz.) Baill.) include schisandrin and gomisin and they have anti-inflammatory and anti-oxidative properties. *In vivo* and *in vitro* studies showed that schisandrin interacted with several inflammatory pathways and inhibited kinase activity, therefore reducing inflammation.[23] Gomisin also reduced inflammation by decreasing the secretion of pro-inflammatory cytokines and inhibiting upstream kinases.[24] In human alveolar epithelial cells and in a lung inflammation mouse model, *wu wei zi* extract reduced nitric oxide (NO) and IL-8 inflammatory mediators. In addition, neutrophil and macrophage infiltration was inhibited and pathological changes in the lung were reduced.[25]

Experimental Studies on xi xin 细辛

Xi xin 细辛 (*Asarum heterotropoides* F. Schm., *Asarum mandshuricum* (Maxim) Kitag.) contains several volatile oils, such as camphene, alpha-pinene, myrcene, sabinene, and limonene.[11] In mice, limonene reduced cytokines (IL-5, IL-13) in BALF and decreased goblet cell metaplasia, thickness of airway smooth muscle, and airway fibrosis, indicating that it can reduce airway remodelling and airway hyper-responsiveness.[26] The compound, zerumbone, from *Zingiber zerumbet*, a species similar to *xi xin*, showed anti-carcinogenic, anti-inflammatory, and anti-oxidant properties.[27] In an asthmatic mouse model, *xi xin* lessened IgE and reduced airway hyperresponsiveness, eosinophils and mucus secretion, and showed an overall anti-allergic effect by regulating Th1/Th2 cytokines.[27]

Experimental Studies on huang qi 黄芪

Huang qi 黄芪 (*Astragalus membranaceus* (Fisch.) Bge., *Astragalus mongholicus* (Bge.) Hsiao) contains the active compounds triterpen-saponins and astragalosides.[8] *Huang qi* lessened airway inflammation, asthma, and allergies in experimental asthma models.[28–30] In one study, IgE decreased as did eosinophils and collagen deposition in the lungs.[28] The *huang qi* compound, astragaloside IV, significantly reduced eosinophils, airway hyperresponsiveness, IL-4 and IL-13 in BALF, and IgE in serum.[29,31] Astragaloside IV also inhibited airway remodelling, smooth muscle hypertrophy, and goblet cell hyperplasia therefore reducing mucous in a murine asthma model.[31] In another study, *huang qi* extract reduced inflammatory cells (eosinophils and lymphocytes) in BALF and airway hyperresponsiveness by reducing allergic cytokines (IL-4, IL-5), and attenuated goblet cell hyperplasia.[30] Together, current research demonstrates that *huang qi* and its constituent compounds have significant bioactive effects on typical asthma inflammation.

Summary of Pharmacological Actions of the Common Herbs

Inflammation appears to be reduced by herbs and their constituent compounds. The effects are largely due to down-regulation of inflammatory mediators and cytokines. Herbs also reduce airway hyperresponsiveness, allergic responses, and oxidative stress. The experimental evidence demonstrates the underlying biochemical actions that contribute to the positive effects seen in asthma clinical trials.

References

1. Ziment I, Tashkin DP. Alternative medicine for allergy and asthma. J Allergy Clin Immunology. 2000;**106**(4):603–14.
2. Ma CH, Ma ZQ, Fu Q, Ma SP. Ma Huang Tang ameliorates asthma through modulation of Th1/Th2 cytokines and inhibition of Th17 cells in ovalbumin-sensitized mice. Chin J Natural Med. 2014;**12**(5):361–6.
3. Asl MN, Hosseinzadeh H. Review of pharmacological effects of Glycyrrhiza sp. and its bioactive compounds. Phytotherapy Research. 2008;**22**(6):709–24.
4. Ma C, Ma Z, Liao XL, Liu J, Fu Q, Ma S. Immunoregulatory effects of glycyrrhizic acid exerts anti-asthmatic effects via modulation of Th1/Th2 cytokines and enhancement of CD4(+)CD25(+)Foxp3+ regulatory T

cells in ovalbumin-sensitized mice. J Ethnopharmacol. 2013;**148**(3): 755–62.

5. Kamei J, Nakamura R, Ichiki H, Kubo M. Antitussive principles of Glycyrrhizae radix, a main component of the Kampo preparations Bakumondo-to (Mai-men-dong-tang). Euro J Pharmacology. 2003;**469**(1–3):159–63.

6. Lim T. Edible Medicinal And Non-Medicinal Plants. Dordrecht: Springer, 2012.

7. Duval C, Auge N, Frisach MF, Casteilla L, Salvayre R, Negre-Salvayre A. Mitochondrial oxidative stress is modulated by oleic acid via an epidermal growth factor receptor-dependent activation of glutathione peroxidase. The Biochemical Journal. 2002;**367**(Pt 3):889–94.

8. Zhou J, Xie G, Yan X. Encyclopedia of Traditional Chinese Medicine: Molecular structures, pharmacological activities, natural sources and applications. Berlin: Springer; 2011.

9. Baskar AA, Al Numair KS, Gabriel Paulraj M, Alsaif MA, Muamar MA, Ignacimuthu S. beta-sitosterol prevents lipid peroxidation and improves anti-oxidant status and histoarchitecture in rats with 1,2-dimethylhydrazine-induced colon cancer. J Med Food. 2012;**15**(4):335–43.

10. Yuk JE, Woo JS, Yun CY, Lee JS, Kim JH, Song GY, *et al.* Effects of lactose-beta-sitosterol and beta-sitosterol on ovalbumin-induced lung inflammation in actively sensitized mice. Int Immunopharmacol. 2007;**7**(12):1517–27.

11. Bensky D, Clavey S, Stoger E. Chinese herbal medicine: Materia medica, 3rd ed. Seattle: Eastland Press; 2004.

12. Chu X, Xu Z, Wu D, Zhao A, Zhou M, Qiu M, *et al. In vitro* and *in vivo* evaluation of the anti-asthmatic activities of fractions from Pheretima. J Ethnopharmacol. 2007;**111**(3):490–5.

13. Balamurugan M, Parthasarathi K, Cooper EL, Ranganathan LS. Anti-inflammatory and anti-pyretic activities of earthworm extract-Lampito mauritii (Kinberg). J Ethnopharmacol. 2009;**121**(2):330–2.

14. Barnes PJ. Drugs for asthma. Br J Pharmacol. 2006 Jan;147 Suppl 1: S297–303.

15. Kim MK, Yoon TY, Choi B. Asthma diagnosis and treatment — 1006. Perillae semen abolished allergic asthmatic response in murine model. World Allergy Organ J. 2013;6 Suppl 1:P6.

16. Deng YM, Xie QM, Zhang SJ, Yao HY, Zhang H. Anti-asthmatic effects of Perilla seed oil in the guinea pig *in vitro* and *in vivo*. Planta medica. 2007;**73**(1):53–8.

17. Okamoto M, Mitsunobu F, Ashida K, Mifune T, Hosaki Y, Tsugeno H, *et al.* Effects of perilla seed oil supplementation on leukotriene generation by leucocytes in patients with asthma associated with lipometabolism. Int Arch Allergy Immunol. 2000;**122**(2):137–42.
18. Yim YK, Lee H, Hong KE, Kim YI, Ko SK, Kim JE, *et al.* Anti-inflammatory and Immune-regulatory Effects of Subcutaneous Perillae Fructus Extract Injections on OVA-induced Asthma in Mice. Evid Based Complement Alternat Med. 2010;**7**(1):79–86.
19. Kang MJ, Ko GS, Oh DG, Kim JS, Noh K, Kang W, *et al.* Role of metabolism by intestinal microbiota in pharmacokinetics of oral baicalin. Arch Pharm Res. 2014;**37**(3):371–8.
20. Lixuan Z, Jingcheng D, Wenqin Y, Jianhua H, Baojun L, Xiaotao F. Baicalin attenuates inflammation by inhibiting NF-κB activation in cigarette smoke induced inflammatory models. Pulm Pharmacol Ther. 2010;**23**(5):411–9.
21. Lucas CD, Dorward DA, Sharma S, Rennie J, Felton JM, Alessandri AL, *et al.* Wogonin Induces Eosinophil Apoptosis and Attenuates Allergic Airway Inflammation. Am J Respir Crit Care Med. 2015;**191**(6):626–36.
22. Kim EH, Shim B, Kang S, Jeong G, Lee Js, Yu YB, *et al.* Anti-inflammatory effects of Scutellaria baicalensis extract via suppression of immune modulators and MAP kinase signaling molecules. J Ethnopharmacol. 2009;**126**(2):320–31.
23. Guo LY, Hung TM, Bae KH, Shin EM, Zhou HY, Hong YN, *et al.* Anti-inflammatory effects of schisandrin isolated from the fruit of Schisandra chinensis Baill. Eur J Pharmacol. 2008;**591**(1–3):293–9.
24. Oh SY, Kim YH, Bae DS, Um BH, Pan CH, Kim CY, *et al.* Anti-inflammatory effects of gomisin N, gomisin J, and schisandrin C isolated from the fruit of Schisandra chinensis. Biosci Biotechnol Biochem. 2010;**74**(2):285–91.
25. Bae H, Kim R, Kim Y, Lee E, Kim HJ, Jang YP, *et al.* Effects of Schisandra chinensis Baillon (Schizandraceae) on lipopolysaccharide induced lung inflammation in mice. J Ethnopharmacol. 2012;**142**(1):41–7.
26. Hirota R, Nakamura H, Bhatti SA, Ngatu NR, Muzembo BA, Dumavibhat N, *et al.* Limonene inhalation reduces allergic airway inflammation in Dermatophagoides farinae-treated mice. Inhal Toxicol. 2012;**24**(6):373–81.
27. Shieh YH, Huang HM, Wang CC, Lee CC, Fan CK, Lee YL. Zerumbone enhances the Th1 response and ameliorates ovalbumin-induced Th2

responses and airway inflammation in mice. Int Immunopharmaccl. 2015;**24**(2):383–91.

28. Chen SM, Tsai YS, Lee SW, Liu YH, Liao SK, Chang WW, *et al*. Astragalus membranaceus modulates Th1/2 immune balance and activates PPARgamma in a murine asthma model. Biochem Cell Biol. 2014;**92**(5):397–405.

29. Huang X, Tang L, Wang F, Song G. Astragaloside IV attenuates allergic inflammation by regulation Th1/Th2 cytokine and enhancement CD4(–) CD25(+)Foxp3 T cells in ovalbumin-induced asthma. Immunobiology. 2014;**219**(7):565–71.

30. Yang ZC, Qu ZH, Yi MJ, Wang C, Ran N, Xie N, *et al*. Astragalus extract attenuates allergic airway inflammation and inhibits nuclear factor kappaB expression in asthmatic mice. Am J Med Sci. 2013;**346**(5):390–5.

31. Du Q, Chen Z, Zhou LF, Zhang Q, Huang M, Yin KS. Inhibitory effec:s of astragaloside IV on ovalbumin-induced chronic experimental asthma. Can J Physiol Pharmacol. 2008;**86**(7):449–57.

7

Clinical Evidence for Acupuncture and Related Therapies

OVERVIEW

Acupuncture has been researched in many clinical studies and this chapter provides an evaluation of the current evidence. Extensive searches of nine scientific databases identified over 20,000 citations of Chinese medicine for adult asthma. They were reviewed against rigorous inclusion criteria, resulting in 49 clinical studies being selected for further analysis. Acupuncture and related therapies improved asthma outcomes in terms of lung function, asthma control, health-related quality of life, and effective rate.

Introduction

Acupuncture and related therapies are used to treat asthma by correcting imbalances and restoring health. Several methods stimulate acupuncture points, some with ancient origins and some more recently developed. Acupuncture therapies include:

- Acupuncture: insertion of an acupuncture needle into acupuncture points on the 14 regular meridians, eight extra meridians, and 48 extra points;
- Electroacupuncture: electrical stimulation of the needle following insertion;
- Moxibustion: application of heat from an ignited material, such as the herb *ai ye* 艾叶, to certain points or areas of the body to induce a warming sensation;
- Acupressure: application of pressure to acupuncture points;

- Scalp acupuncture: application of micro-system acupuncture on the scalp;
- Acupoint magnet therapy: application of a magnetic force to acupuncture points;
- Laser acupuncture: application of laser irradiation to acupuncture points.

Included studies are indicated by an "A" followed by a number, e.g. (A1). The reference list for included studies can be found at the end of this chapter.

Previous Systematic Reviews

Acupuncture treatment for asthma has received considerable research attention over the past 30 years. Recently, systematic reviews have covered topics such as heat-sensitive moxibustion[1] and needle acupuncture for asthma.[2] In a review of heat-sensitive moxibustion, 14 randomised controlled trials (RCTs) were analysed.[1] Results showed improved effective rates but not asthma control measured with the Asthma Control Test (ACT) or lung function. The authors concluded that heat-sensitive moxibustion did not improve asthma compared to routine pharmacotherapy and suggested that higher-quality RCTs are needed to fully understand its effects. A Cochrane review published in 2003 and updated in 2008 reported results from 12 RCTs.[2] The authors found that not enough evidence was available to conclude if acupuncture should be recommended, and suggested that further research is needed. New research has become available since these systematic reviews. In this chapter, new research as well as older studies are evaluated and the results are pooled in a meta-analysis.

Characteristics of Clinical Studies of Acupuncture and Related Therapies

Database searches identified a total of 28,153 citations. After removal of duplicates, 18,684 were screened and 1,429 had full-text review. After exclusions, 36 RCTs and 13 non-controlled studies were included (Figure 7.1).

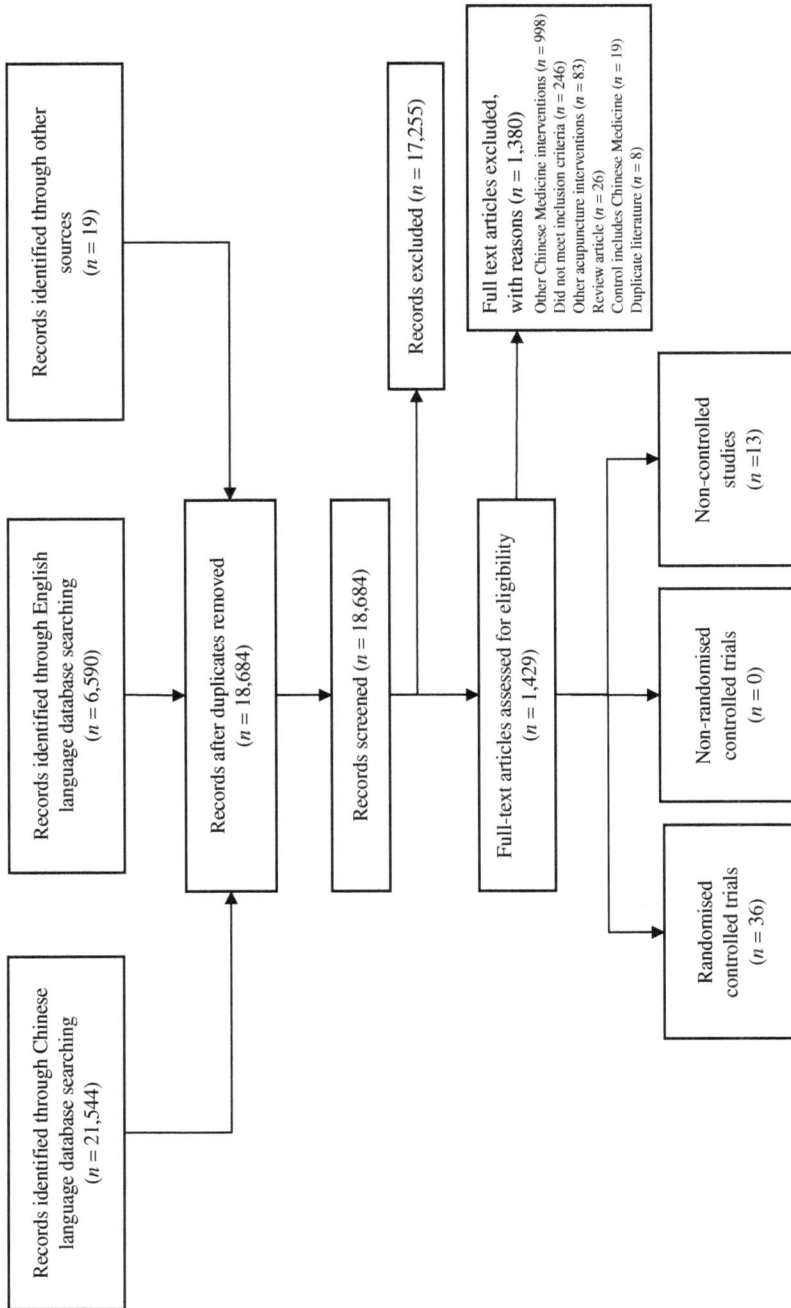

Figure 7.1 Flow chart of study selection process: acupuncture and related therapies.

Most research was conducted in mainland China, but one study was conducted in each of the following countries: UK, Korea, Taiwan, Brazil, Switzerland, New Zealand, Iran, Israel, and Australia. Findings from controlled clinical trials are pooled in the current meta-analysis to provide evidence for acupuncture therapies. Non-controlled studies are summarised but their results are not included in the evidence analysis.

Eleven different acupuncture therapies were documented in the included studies:

- Acupuncture (n = 18);
- Moxibustion (n = 18);
- Laser acupuncture (n = 3);
- Electroacupuncture (n = 2);
- Ultrasonic leading (n = 2);
- Acupoint magnet therapy (n = 1);
- Acupressure (n = 1);
- Ear acupressure (n = 1);
- Hot compress acupressure (n = 1);
- Scalp acupuncture (n = 1);
- Transcutaneous electrical nerve stimulation (TENS) acupuncture (n = 1).

Most of these therapies have been used throughout Chinese medicine (CM) history. However, others, such as ear acupuncture and scalp acupuncture, have emerged as new techniques in the last century. Laser acupuncture, electroacupuncture, ultrasonic leading, magnet therapy, and TENS have also emerged as new technologies incorporated into CM practice.

The most common acupuncture points across all types of acupuncture interventions were BL13 *Feishu* 肺俞 (30 studies), EX-B1 *Dingchuan* 定喘 (18 studies), ST36 *Zusanli* 足三里 (12 studies), and CV22 *Tiantu* 天突 (9 studies). CM syndromes included Lung, Spleen, and Kidney deficiency, wind-cold, wind-heat, phlegm, and Blood stasis. A summary of the studies is presented in Table 7.1.

Table 7.1 Summary of all Acupuncture and Related Therapies in Clinical Studies

No. of Studies	No. of Participants	Most Common Syndromes (No. of Studies)	Most Common Acupuncture Points (No. of Studies)
49	3,310	Lung, Spleen, and Kidney deficiency (2)	BL13 Feishu 肺俞 (30)
		wind-cold, wind-heat or phlegm (2)	EX-B1 Dingchuan 定喘 (18)
		Phlegm-cold (1)	ST36 Zusanli 足三里 (12)
		Kidney deficiency (1)	CV22 Tiantu 天突 (9)
		Lung and Kidney deficiency and Blood stasis (1)	BL20 Pishu 脾俞 (8)
		Spleen deficiency (1)	CV17 Danzhong 膻中 (8)
			GV14 Dazhui 大椎 (8)
			LI4 Hegu 合谷 (8)
			LU6 Kongzui 孔最 (8)
			ST40 Fenglong 丰隆 (8)
			LI11 Quchi 曲池 (7)
			LU10 Yuji 鱼际 (7)
			LU7 Lieque 列缺 (7)
			BL23 Shenshu 肾俞 (6)
			LU5 Chize 尺泽 (5)
			LU9 Taiyuan 太渊 (5)
			CV12 Zhongwan 中脘 (4)
			LU1 Zhongfu 中府 (4)
			PC6 Neiguan 内关 (4)

Randomised Controlled Trials of Acupuncture and Related Therapies

Acupuncture has been evaluated in 36 RCTs including 2,855 participants (A1–A36). Chronic asthma was evaluated in 30 studies and acute asthma in six studies (Table 7.2). All participants were diagnosed with asthma according to internationally recognised definitions such as those in the Global Initiative for Asthma (GINA) guidelines. Duration of asthma ranged from six months to 40 years. Participants' age ranged from 17 to 85 years old. There were similar numbers of male and female patients, 1,068 and 1,114 respectively (gender not stated for 673 participants). CM syndromes were described in five studies. Syndromes included Lung, Spleen, and Kidney deficiency and wind-cold, wind-heat or phlegm.

Table 7.2 Summary of Acupuncture and Related Therapies in Clinical Studies: Randomised Controlled Trials

Asthma Stage	No. of Studies	No. of Participants	Most Common Syndromes (No. of Studies)	Most Common Acupuncture Points (No. of Studies)
Acute	6	448	Lung, Spleen, and Kidney deficiency (n = 1)	BL13 Feishu 肺俞 (4) EX-B1 Dingchuan 定喘 (3) CV17 Danzhong 膻中 (2) CV22 Tiantu 天突 (2) GV14 Dazhui 大椎 (2) LU6 Kongzui 孔最 (2) All other acupuncture points were used in one study.
Chronic	30	2,407	wind-cold, wind-heat or phlegm (n = 2) Lung, Spleen, and Kidney deficiency (n = 1) Phlegm-Cold (n = 1) Kidney deficiency (n = 1) Lung and Kidney deficiency and Blood stasis (n = 1) Spleen deficiency (n = 1)	BL13 Feishu 肺俞 (16) EX-B1 Dingchuan 定喘 (9) ST36 Zusanli 足三里 (7) LU10 Yuji 鱼际 (6) LU6 Kongzui 孔最 (6) BL20 Pishu 脾俞 (5) BL23 Shenshu 肾俞 (5) CV17 Danzhong 膻中 (5) LI11 Quchi 曲池 (5) LI4 Hegu 合谷 (5) LU5 Chize 尺泽 (5) LU7 Lieque 列缺 (5) All other acupuncture points were used in four or fewer studies.

Acupuncture treatments were separated into nine categories:

- Acupuncture (14 studies);
- Moxibustion (14 studies);
- Electroacupuncture (two studies);

- Acupressure (one study);
- Ear acupressure (one study);
- Acupoint magnet therapy (one study);
- Hot compress acupressure (one study);
- Laser acupuncture (one study);
- Scalp acupuncture (one study).

The most commonly reported acupuncture points were BL13 *Feishu* 肺俞 and EX-B1 *Dingchuan* 定喘 (Table 7.2). Treatment duration ranged between one day and three years. Comparators included pharmacotherapy (n = 26), sham or placebo acupuncture (n = 10), or no treatment (n = two). Pharmacotherapies included bronchodilators (salbutamol, theophylline) and/or corticosteroids (budesonide, fluticasone) and their combinations.

Risk of Bias

All 36 RCTs were described as randomised and methods for sequence generation and allocation concealment were described in five studies (A16, A18, A25–A27). Blinding of participants with placebo treatments or sham acupuncture was described in nine studies (A1–A3, A5–A8, A15, A35). Blinding of personnel was not possible in the majority of studies because acupuncture therapy needs to be performed by a qualified professional. All studies therefore suffered high bias risk with regards to personnel blinding. Outcome assessors were blind in eight studies. Incomplete outcome data was mostly at low risk of bias because the drop-out rate was small and balanced between groups. Selective outcome reporting was judged to carry unclear risk of bias for most studies because published protocols were not available. The overall methodological quality of the studies was low (Table 7.3).

Acupuncture

Ten studies used acupuncture as the intervention and four used acupuncture combined with routine pharmacotherapy. These studies included a total of 1,057 participants (A1–A14). All studies evaluated

Table 7.3   Risk of Bias of RCTs: Acupuncture and Related Therapies

Risk of Bias Domain	Low Risk n (%)	Unclear Risk n (%)	High Risk n (%)
Sequence generation	14 (38.9%)	21 (58.3%)	1 (2.8%)
Allocation concealment	6 (16.7%)	29 (80.6%)	1 (2.8%)
Blinding of participants	9 (25.0%)	1 (2.8%)	26 (72.2%)
Blinding of personnel*	0	1 (2.8%)	35 (97.2%)
Blinding of outcome assessors	8 (22.2%)	9 (25.0%)	19 (52.8%)
Incomplete outcome data	30 (83.3%)	4 (11.1%)	2 (5.6%)
Selective outcome reporting	0	34 (94.4%)	2 (5.6%)

*Blinding of personnel (acupuncturists) is virtually impossible in manual therapy studies.

participants with chronic asthma except for one that assessed acute asthma (A9). Two studies reported that participants had pathogenic wind-cold, wind-heat, or phlegm, and two studies reported either Lung and Spleen deficiency or Lung, Spleen, and Kidney deficiency. BL13 *Feishu* 肺俞 (10 studies), EX-B1 *Dingchuan* 定喘 (six studies), LU10 *Yuji* 鱼际 (five studies), and LU6 *Kongzui* 孔最 (five studies) were the most frequently reported acupuncture points.

Effects of the Intervention: Acupuncture

Acupuncture compared with sham acupuncture did not improve forced expiratory volume in one second (FEV_1L) (mean difference (MD) 0.22 –0.01, 0.46], I^2 = 0%) (A2–A3) but did improve lung function FEV_1% predicted by 3.14% [1.27, 5.01], I^2 = 0% (A6–A8). Other outcomes, such as peak expiratory flow (PEF) L/s (MD 0.89 [–0.34, 2.12], and rescue medication usage, (MD –1.40 [–414, 1.34]) could only be evaluated in single studies and results did not show a statistically significant difference between acupuncture and sham acupuncture or pharmacotherapy. Results from a single study suggested acupuncture plus salbutamol resulted in clinically and statistically significant improvements in quality of life compared with salbutamol alone (MD 30.10 points on the Asthma Quality of Life Questionnaire (AQLQ) scale [11.79, 54.41] (A1). For acute asthma, acupuncture plus pharmacotherapy improved the chance of achieving a clinical improvement by 1.32 times that of pharmacotherapy alone [1.06, 1.63] based on the Chinese Medicine Clinical Research Guidelines (A10).

Acupuncture appears to be well tolerated by people with asthma. Eight mild adverse events were reported in five studies (A2, A6, A8, A11, A13). Events included pain at acupuncture points (two cases), itching (two cases), dizziness (one case), nausea/vomiting (one case), exacerbation of asthma (one case), and infection (one case).

Electroacupuncture

Two studies used electroacupuncture to treat acute or chronic asthma (A15–A16). Compared with theophylline, there was no difference between intervention and control groups in terms of $FEV_1\%$ (MD 1.70 [–8.15, 11.55]), PEF L/s (MD 0.02 [–0.14, 0.18]), use of rescue medication (MD 0.66 [–1.53, 2.85]), or effective rate (RR 1.08 [–0.90, 1.30]). Studies did not report adverse events.

Assessment Using GRADE: Acupuncture

The main comparison of acupuncture against sham acupuncture for chronic asthma is presented in a Grading of Recommendations Assessment, Development and Evaluation (GRADE) summary of findings table. The quality of evidence for acupuncture versus sham acupuncture was moderate (Table 7.4). The result was statistically significant for $FEV_1\%$, but not significant for PEF L/s, rescue bronchodilator use, and quality of life. Asthma control and exacerbation frequency were not measured.

Moxibustion

Moxibustion was evaluated in 14 studies (A17–A30). Eight studies used moxibustion at specific acupuncture points, commonly BL13 *Feishu* 肺俞 and ST36 *Zusanli* 足三里 (A18, A21–A25, A28, A30). Seven studies applied moxibustion over a meridian area including the Bladder and Governor Vessel (A17, A19–A20, A26–A27, A29–A30).

Table 7.4   GRADE: Acupuncture vs. Sham Acupuncture for Chronic Asthma

Outcomes and Follow-up	No. of Participants (Studies)	Quality of the Evidence (GRADE)	Relative Effect (95% CI)	Anticipated Absolute Effects	
				Risk with Sham-Acupuncture	Risk Difference with Acupuncture
Lung function: FEV_1 % Treatment duration: mean 2.5 weeks	84 (2 RCTs)	⊕⊕⊕◯ MODERATE[1]	—	The mean FEV_1 in the control group was **78.8%**	MD **3.14 higher** (1.27 higher to 5.01 higher)
Lung function: PEF L/s Treatment duration: 4 weeks	30 (1 RCT)	⊕⊕⊕◯ MODERATE[1]	—	The mean PEF in the control group was **4.5 L/s**	MD **0.89 higher** (0.34 lower to 2.12 higher)
Use of rescue medication: Weekly usage Treatment duration: 1 week	26 (1 RCT)	⊕⊕⊕◯ MODERATE[1]	—	The mean rescue bronchodilator use in the control group was **8.1 puffs**	MD **1.4 lower** (4.14 lower to 1.34 higher)
Quality of life: AQLQ[2] Treatment duration: 2 weeks	44 (1 RCT)	⊕⊕⊕◯ MODERATE[1]	—	The mean AQLQ in the control group was **158 points**	MD **11 lower** (32.6 lower to 10.6 higher)

Asthma control and exacerbation frequency — not reported

Adverse events

Three studies reported adverse events. Events in intervention groups included pain at the site of acupuncture (2 cases), nausea and/or vomiting (1 case), exacerbation of asthma (1 case), and lung infection (1 case). Adverse events in control groups included exacerbation of asthma (2 cases) (A2, A6, A8).

NB. The risk in the intervention group (and its 95% CI) is based on the assumed risk in the comparison group and the relative effect of the intervention (and its 95% CI).

Abbreviations: AQLQ, Asthma Quality of Life Questionnaire; Confidence interval; FEV1, Forced Effective Volume; GRADE, Grading of Recommendations Assessment, Development and Evaluation; FEV$_1$, Forced Expiratory Volume in One Second; MD: Mean Difference; PEF, Peak Expiratory Flow; RCT, Randomised Controlled Trial.

Notes:

1. Small sample size limits certainty of results.
2. AQLQ: 32 items, range: 32–224 points. Higher scores indicate better quality of life.

Study References:

- Lung function (FEV$_1$ %): A6, A8
- Lung function (PEF L/s): A2
- Use of rescue medication: A8
- Quality of life: A1

Moxibustion techniques included needle head moxa, indirect moxa, and thermal moxa. Thermal moxa is a relatively new technique but is similar to the traditional style for the purposes of clinical trial analysis. Comparators were pharmacotherapy in all studies. Duration of treatment ranged from one month to three months. Participants had Spleen deficiency in one study and Kidney deficiency in the other (A23, A29).

Effects of the Intervention: Moxibustion

Moxibustion compared with routine pharmacotherapy for chronic asthma statistically improved lung function $FEV_1\%$ predicted by an average of 3% ([0.75, 5.25], I^2 = 17%) (Table 7.9). In these studies, moxibustion was commonly applied to the Bladder meridian between BL13 *Feishu* 肺俞 to BL17 *Geshu* 膈俞. Moxibustion did not produce statistically significant improvements in PEF% (MD 1.67 [–4.28, 7.62], I^2 = 42%). The ACT (MD 0.45 [–0.10, 1.00], I^2 = 10%) and total effective rate (RR 1.06 [0.81, 1.38], I^2 = 37%) were not improved by moxibustion compared to pharmacotherapy (Table 7.5).

Adverse events such as headaches (five cases) and palpitations (four cases) were reported after treatment (A20). Two studies reported no events and the remaining studies did not mention if adverse events had occurred (A17, A28).

Acupressure

Two studies assessed patients with acute asthma. Of these, one used acupressure on body points (A31) and the other used a hot compress of herbs (A32). Another study used ear acupressure for chronic asthma (A33).

Body acupressure on CV22 *Tiantu* 天突, EX-B1 *Dingchuan* 定喘, BL13 *Feishu* 肺俞, CV17 *Danzhong* 膻中, and GV14 *Dazhui* 大椎 was applied for two weeks and the treatment outcomes were compared with salbutamol treatment (A31). The results showed that lung function improved (FEV_1 L 0.48 L [0.30, 0.66], $FEV_1\%$ 8.08% [6.98, 9.18], PEF L/s 0.76 [0.37, 1.15], and PEF% 7.20% [1.58, 12.82], but the effective rate did not (RR 1.07 [0.96, 1.20]; (A31). Hot compress of herbs plus

Table 7.5   Moxibustion

Comparator	Outcome	No. of Studies	No. of Participants	Effect Size MD/RR [95% CI]	I² %	Included Studies
Pharmacotherapy	FEV₁ %	6	610	3.00 [0.75, 5.25]*	17	S17, 19–20, 24–25, 27
Pharmacotherapy	PEF%	3	135	1.67 [–4.28, 7.62]	42	S17, 24, 27
Pharmacotherapy	Eff. Rate Bronchial Asthma Guide	2	102	1.06 [0.81, 1.38]	37	S17, 19
Pharmacotherapy	ACT	3	398	0.45 [–0.10, 1.00]	18	S19–20, 26

*Statistically significant.

Abbreviations: ACT, Asthma Control Test; CI, Confidence Interval; FEV₁, Forced Expiratory Volume in One Second; MD, Mean Difference; PEF, Peak Expiratory Flow.

pharmacotherapy compared to pharmacotherapy alone did not improve FEV_1 L (MD 0.00 L [–0.21, 0.21]) but did improve effective rate (risk ratio RR 1.12 [1.02, 1.24]) (A32).

Ear acupressure compared to placebo ear acupressure for 60 days improved participants' ACT score by 1.8 points [0.14, 3.46] but did not improve FEV_1% (MD 3.03 [–0.29, 6.35]) (A33). Adverse events were reported in the ear acupressure study where two participants from the intervention group and one from the control group experienced cases of contact dermatitis (A33).

Acupoint Magnet Therapy

Magnets were placed on BL13 *Feishu* 肺俞, BL23 *Shenshu* 肾俞, and CV17 *Danzhong* 膻中 for three days every January for three years in one study (A34). Acupoint magnet therapy plus salbutamol compared to salbutamol alone showed small increases in lung function according to FEV_1 L (MD 0.33 L [0.19, 0.47]) and PEF (MD 0.73 L's [0.26, 1.20]) but not forced vital capacity litres. Effective rate was improved by 1.15 times that of salbutamol based on the Chinese Medicine Clinical Research Guidelines [1.04, 1.27] (A34). Adverse events were not reported in this study.

Laser Acupuncture

One study compared laser acupuncture with sham laser acupuncture (non-specific points) (A35). Treatment was given for five weeks followed by three weeks of washing-out, before participants were crossed over for another five weeks. The results were not presented in a way that could allow analysis and interpretation. Adverse events were not reported in this study.

Scalp Acupuncture

One study used scalp acupuncture compared with terbutalin for 10 days (A36). There was no difference in FEV_1 L (MD 0.13 [−0.24, 0.503]); or PEF L/s (MD 0.18 [−0.75, 1.11]) between groups. The study did not report adverse events.

Frequently Reported Acupuncture Points in Meta-analyses Showing Favourable Effect

The most frequently used acupuncture points in meta-analyses showing favourable effect were calculated according to outcome category and intervention type. Table 7.6 includes the full list of acupuncture points.

Controlled Clinical Trails of Acupunture and Related Therapies

Controlled Clinical trials were not found.

Non-controlled Studies of Acupuncture and Related Therapies

A total of 13 case series consisting of 455 participants were included (A37–A49). Although the characteristics of these non-controlled studies were evaluated, results were not assessed due to the high number

Table 7.6 Frequently Reported Acupuncture Points in Meta-analyses Showing Favourable Effect

Intervention	Outcome Category	No. of Meta-analyses	No. Studies in Meta-analyses	Acupuncture Points (No. of Studies)
Acupuncture vs. sham/ placebo	Lung function	1	2	GV14 Dazhui 大椎 (1)
				EX-B1 Dingchuan 定喘 (1)
				BL13 Feishu 肺俞 (1)
				KI3 Taixi 太溪 (1)
				LU10 Yuji 鱼际 (1)
				SP6 Sanyinjiao 三阴交 (1)
				LI4 Hegu 合谷 (1)
				LI11 Quchi 曲池 (1)
				ST36 Zusanli 足三里 (1)
				LR13 Zhangmen 章门 (1)
				PC6 Neiguan 内关 (1)
Moxibustion vs. drug(s)	Lung function	1	6	BL13 肺俞-BL17 (4)
				LI20 Yingxiang 迎香 (1)
				ST36 Zusanli 足三里 (1)
				LU5 Chize 尺泽 (1)
				LU6 Kongzui 孔最 (1)
				LU10 Yuji 鱼际 (1)
				LU7 Lieque 列缺 (1)

Frequently reported acupuncture points in meta-analyses showing favourable effect are calculated by selecting the effective pools for each outcome category based on the intervention type. The acupuncture points used in the individual studies are then counted. Pools are considered to be effective if they show a statistically significant effect at end of treatment between groups.

of randomised controlled trials contributing better quality evidence. CM syndromes were reported in four studies and common syndromes included phlegm-cold and Lung, Spleen, and Kidney deficiency (A37–A38, A42, A48). Acupuncture therapies included needle acupuncture (four studies), moxibustion (four studies), laser acupuncture (four studies), ultrasonic leading (two studies), and TENS acupuncture (one study). The most common acupuncture points in non-controlled studies were BL13 *Feishu* 肺俞 (nine studies), EX-B1 *Dingchuan* 定喘 (six studies), ST36 *Zusanli* 足三里 (four studies), ST40 *Fenglong* 丰隆 (four studies), BL20 *Pishu* 脾俞 (three studies),

GV14 *Dazhui* 大椎 (three studies), and CV22 *Tiantu* 天突 (three studies). Other points were used in fewer than three studies. One study (A37) reported adverse events, specifically red skin and itching after ultrasonic leading at BL13 *Feishu* 肺俞. The other studies did not report if adverse events occurred.

Summary of Acupuncture and Related Therapies Clinical Evidence

Acupuncture and related therapies led to improvements in various aspects of asthma, including lung function, asthma control, quality of life, and total effective rate. Lung function was improved by acupuncture and moxibustion during acute exacerbations and chronic asthma.

Acupuncture showed the greatest improvement in total effective rate when combined with pharmacotherapy compared with pharmacotherapy alone. Other interventions such as moxibustion did not improve total effective rate. Other outcomes such as quality of life, rescue medication, and exacerbation frequency were seldom used in the included studies and could not be pooled for analysis. Sub-groups according to duration of treatment and duration of asthma could not be analysed due to the small number of studies in each meta-analysis. Other therapies such as acupressure and scalp acupuncture did not produce a result greater than control interventions.

Overall, few adverse events were reported and acupuncture therapies appear to be well tolerated by people with asthma. Most of the studies did not include details about CM syndromes. In the studies that did report syndromes, Lung, Spleen, and Kidney deficiency was common, as was phlegm-cold, phlegm-heat, and phlegm blocking the Lungs. The most common acupuncture points across all studies were BL13 *Feishu* 肺俞, EX-B1 *Dingchuan* 定喘, ST36 *Zusanli* 足三里, and CV22 *Tiantu* 天突. These points were found to be consistently effective in meta-analyses demonstrating positive effects.

Acupuncture and related therapies can improve outcomes for patients suffering from chronic asthma and acute exacerbations of asthma. These improvements were statistically significant but in most cases did not meet the clinically meaningful amount. Acupuncture and related therapies appear safe for people with asthma and may be considered for use in clinical practice.

References

1. Xiong J, Liu Z, Chen R, Xie D, Chi Z, Zhang B. Effectiveness and safety of Heat-sensitive moxibustion on bronchial asthma: a meta-analysis of randomized control trials. J Tradit Chin Med. 2014;**34**(4):392–400.
2. McCarney RW, Brinkhaus B, Lasserson TJ, Linde K. Acupuncture for chronic asthma. Cochrane Database Syst Rev. 2004;CD000008.

References to Included Acupunture and Related Therapies Studies

Study No.	Reference
A1	Biernacki WP, M. D. Acupuncture in treatment of stable asthma. Resp Med 1998; 92(9):1143–5.
A2	Choi JYJ, Kim HJ, Lee JI, Kang MS, Roh KW, Choi YL, *et al*. A randomized pilot study of acupuncture as an adjunct therapy in adult asthmatic patients. *J Asthma* 2010;47(7):774–80.
A3	Chu KA, Wu YC, Ting YM, Wang HC, Lu JY. Acupuncture therapy results in immediate bronchodilating effect in asthma patients. Journal of the Chinese Medical Association: *JCMA* 2007;70(7):265–8.
A4	Lai X. Observation on the curative effect of acupuncture on type I allergic diseases. *J Tradit Chin Med* 1993 Dec;13(4):243–8.
A5	Lin CA, Pai HJ, Almeida FM, Saraiva-Romanholo BM, Martins MA.Effects of acupuncture in spirometry and quality of life in mild and moderate asthma patients [Abstract]. American Thoracic Society International Conference, May 15–20, 2009, San Diego. 2012:A1285.

(*Continued*)

(*Continued*)

Study No.	Reference
A6	Medici TC, Grebski E, Wu J, Hinz G, Wuthrich B. Acupuncture and bronchial asthma: a long-term randomized study of the effects of real versus sham acupuncture compared to controls in patients with bronchial asthma. *J Alt Compl Med* 2002;8(6):737–50
A7	Mitchell P, Wells JE. E. Acupuncture for chronic asthma: a controlled trial with six months follow-up. *Am J Acupunct* 1989;17(1):5–13
A8	Shapira MY, Berkman N, Ben-David G, Avital A, Bardach E, Breuer R. Short-term acupuncture therapy is of no benefit in patients with moderate persistent asthma. *Chest* 2002;121(5):1396–400
A9	Fu WB, Chen XH, Chen QX. Clinical observation of eye acupuncture in treating acute attack of asthma. *J Acupunct Tuina Sci* 2005;3(3):10–2
A10	贾钧, 周立云, 林静. 穴位针刺治疗缓解期支气管哮喘 48 例临床观察. 河北中医. 2013,35(10):1524–1525
A11	谭程, 张昶, 高丹, 等. 从肺肠论治针刺对支气管哮喘患者生命质量的影响. 中国针灸. 2012,32(8): 673–677
A12	雷建华, 刘金阁. 自血穴位注射治疗支气管哮喘的临床观察. 河北中医. 2008,30(4):367–368
A13	付钰, 张昶, 王宝凯, 等. 针刺从肺肠论治对支气管哮喘患者中医症状的影响. 北京中医药大学学报. 2013,36(4):272–276
A14	张梦, 洪嘉婧, 洪杰, 等. 降气平喘针法治疗哮喘随机对照临床研究. 长春中医药大学学报. 2012,28(4):603–604
A15	Najafizadeh K, Vosughian M, Rasaian N, Sohrabpour H, Deilami MD, Ghadiani M, *et al.* A randomized double blind placebo controlled trial on the short and long term effects of electro acupuncture on moderate to severe asthma. *Euro Resp J* 2006; 28(Suppl 50):502s [E2897].
A16	李巍, 谭洛, 苗林艳, 等. 电针肺俞穴对支气管哮喘患者 (急性发作期) 临床症状与肺功能的影响. 针灸临床杂志. 2010,26(01):4–8
A17	杨坤. 腧穴热敏化艾灸治疗慢性持续期支气管哮喘的临床研究[D]. 武汉: 湖北中医药大学, 2010
A18	杨进荣. 针刺结合温和灸三俞穴治疗支气管哮喘 56 例临床研究[D]. 广州: 广州中医药大学, 2006
A19	欧阳八四, 高洁, 孙钢, 等. 热敏灸对慢性持续期支气管哮喘患者肺功能和生活质量的影响: 随机对照研究. 中国针灸. 2011,31(11):965–970

(*Continued*)

(Continued)

Study No.	Reference
A20	Chen RC, Xiong M, Chi J, Zhang Z, Tian B, Xu N, *et al.* Curative effect of heat-sensitive moxibustion on chronic persistent asthma: a multicenter randomized controlled trial. Journal of traditional Chinese medicine. *J Trad Chin Med* 2014; 33(5):584–91
A21	艾瑞东, 王雅娟. 隔姜灸联合针刺法治疗支气管哮喘缓解期 30 例临床观察. 河北中医. 2011,33(5):742–743
A22	周一兰. 壮医药线点灸加氨茶碱治疗支气管哮喘 30 例临床观察. 广西中医药. 2012,35(4):47–48
A23	吴兆利, 刘自力. 培土生金法针灸治疗支气管哮喘 35 例观察. 实用中医内科杂志. 2007,21(2):4–5
A24	郑美凤, 罗彩云, 何芙蓉. 补土通窍针法对变应性鼻炎-哮喘综合征患者肺功能的影响. 福建中医药大学学报. 2012,22(2):17–19
A25	孙冬梅, 杨进荣, 刘坛树, 等. 温和灸三俞穴结合针刺治疗支气管哮喘临床研究. 新中医. 2012,44(5):102–103
A26	宋南昌, 何金保, 徐涵斌, 等. 热敏灸与舒利迭治疗支气管哮喘慢性持续期的比较研究. 中国针灸. 2012,32(7):593–596
A27	梁超, 张唐法,杨坤. 腧穴热敏灸与西药治疗慢性持续期支气管哮喘疗效对照观察. 中国针灸. 2010,30(11):886–890
A28	李蓉, 刘耀, 彭晓虹, 等. 灼灸对支气管哮喘慢性持续期临床疗效及IgE的影响研究. 现代临床医学. 2012,38(2):100–102
A29	鲍鑫宇, 周庆伟, 钱航. 督灸联合西医常规治疗肺肾气虚型缓解期哮喘 30 例. 中医研究. 2013,26(7):66–68
A30	梁超, 黄国付, 杨坤, 等. 腧穴热敏灸对慢性持续期哮喘肺功能近远期影响. 中国康复. 2010,25(4):275–276
A31	干丽萍, 涂长英. 穴位按摩与 β2-受体激动剂治疗支气管哮喘的疗效. 实用临床医学. 2013,14(1):10–11
A32	杨美艳, 何良文, 罗华泰, 等. 自拟化痰定喘散热敷佐治支气管哮喘 75 例临床观察. 疑难病杂志. 2009,8(3):162–163
A33	罗胜, 李俊雄, 凌孟晖. 耳穴压贴治疗哮喘慢性持续期的临床疗效观察. 中医临床研究. 2013,5(7):43–45
A34	才江平, 冯燕, 曲娜, 等. 复方沙丁胺醇、联合咳喘磁疗贴治疗支气管哮喘的临床研究 (附80例病例). 中国民族民间医药. 2010:145–146
A35	Tandon MK, Soh PF, Wood AT. Acupuncture for bronchial asthma? A double-blind crossover study. *MJA* 1991; 154(6):409–12

(Continued)

(Continued)

Study No.	Reference
A36	刘智斌, 牛文民. 头皮发际区微针法治疗支气管哮喘 28 例. 现代中医药. 2008,28(5):69–70
A37	王微. 温肺化饮散经肺腧靶向给药对支气管哮喘（寒哮证）肺功能及生化指标影响的临床研究. 新中医. 2005;37(12):26–7
A38	赵吉平 崔. 温和灸治疗支气管哮喘缓解期 36 例疗效观察. 中国民间疗法. 2002;10(4):21
A39	张静 章, 赵玉霞,. 三伏艾灸预防支气管哮喘发作 63 例临床研究. 江苏中医药. 2009;41(3):53–4
A40	丛天竹. 针刺为主治疗支气管哮喘 30 例疗效观察. 航空航天医药. 2010;(6):1059
A41	安茂国. 虚寒性哮喘腧穴艾炷灸治疗效果的临床观察. 中国医药指南. 2011;9(31):377–8
A42	汪世全. 中西医结合治疗顽固性哮喘38例. 安徽医学. 1998;(04):80
A43	葛通远阎奕莹张桂珠. 激光治疗支气管哮喘中免疫效应的探讨. 哈尔滨医药. 1982;(03):133–5
A44	葛通远闫奕莹张桂林. 激光治疗支气管哮喘中免疫效应的探讨. 激光. 1980;(10):57
A45	方针. 五穴灸治疗支气管哮喘. 云南中医杂志. 1991;(05):29
A46	马淑骅 陈. 支气管哮喘(缓解期)患者背部热敏腧穴分布的临床研究. 江西中医药. 2011;42(1):30–2
A47	Chu KA, Wu YC, Lin MH, Wang HC. Acupuncture resulting in immediate bronchodilating response in asthma patients. *J Chin Med Assoc* 2005;68(12):591–4
A48	Hu J. Clinical observation on 25 cases of hormone dependent bronchial asthma treated by acupuncture. *J Trad Chin Med* 1998 Mar;18(1):27–30
A49	Sovijärvi AR, Poppius H. Acute bronchodilating effect of transcutaneous nerve stimulation in asthma. A peripheral reflex or psychogenic response. *Scand J Respir Dis* 1977; 58(3):164–9

8

Clinical Evidence for Other Chinese Medicine Therapies

OVERVIEW

Other Chinese medicine therapies include *qigong* 气功, *tuina* 推拿, and cupping. These therapies have been evaluated in clinical studies. This chapter provides an evaluation of the current clinical trial literature and summarises the evidence of these therapies for asthma. Comprehensive searches of nine databases identified more than 20,000 citations. Rigorous inclusion criteria were applied and a total of six clinical studies were included.

Introduction

In addition to Chinese herbal medicine (CHM) and acupuncture therapies, Chinese medicine (CM) includes a range of other therapies to treat disease and maintain health. These include:

- Cupping therapy: application of suction by placing a vaccumised cup onto the body;
- *Tuina* 推拿: Chinese massage therapy;
- *Qigong* 气功: Chinese physical exercises and breathing techniques.

Included studies are indicated by an "O" followed by a number, e.g. (O1). The reference list for included studies can be found at the end of this chapter.

Previous Systematic Reviews

A systematic review reported that *tai chi* 太极 is an effective therapy for asthma.[1] Only one asthma study was included in this review and the other studies evaluated chronic obstructive pulmonary disease. The asthma study evaluated children and reported that after 12 weeks, those in the treatment groups showed improved forced expiratory volume in one second (FEV_1), forced vital capacity (FVC), and peak expiratory flow (PEF) versus the control group.[1] In another review, Cao *et al*. showed that cupping therapy can potentially benefit patients suffering from asthma as well as pain and other conditions. However, these studies were evaluated separately and statistical evaluation was not performed.[2]

Characteristics of Clinical Studies of Other Chinese Medicine Therapies

Electronic searches in nine databases found a total of 28,153 citations. Of these, 18,684 were screened and 1,429 were subject to full-text review. One randomised controlled trial and five non-controlled studies including 272 participants were included (Fig. 8.1). Therapies included cupping, *tuina* 推拿, and *qigong* 气功.

Randomised Controlled Trials of Other Chinese Medicine Therapies

One randomised controlled trial (RCT) with 136 participants used cupping to treat asthma (O1). The mean age of participants was 43.98 years. Males accounted for 61 participants and females 75 participants. Cupping plus routine pharmacotherapy was compared to routine pharmacotherapy alone. Cupping was administered three times a week for four weeks and cups were retained for 5–10 minutes each time (O1). CM syndromes were not reported in the study.

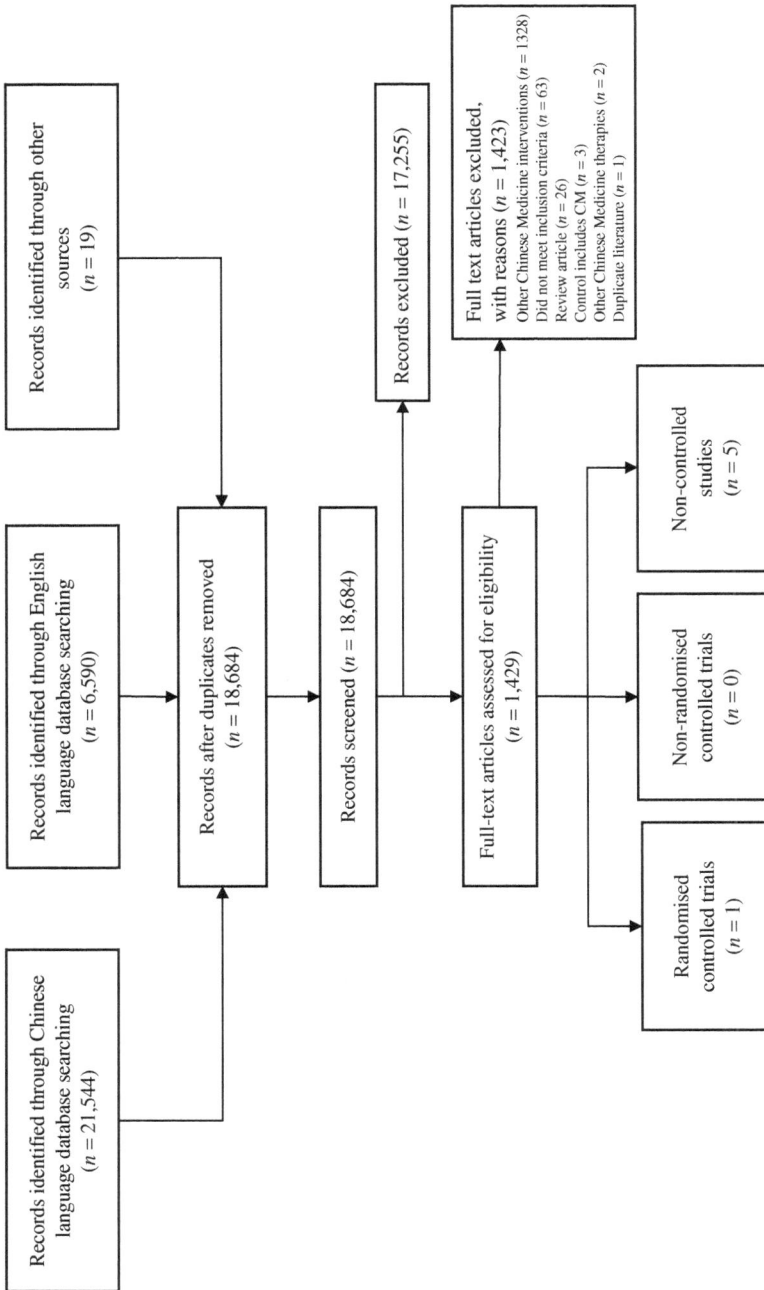

Figure 8.1 Flow chart of study selection process: other Chinese medicine therapies.

Records identified through other sources
($n = 19$)

Records identified through English language database searching
($n = 6,590$)

Records identified through Chinese language database searching
($n = 21,544$)

Records after duplicates removed
($n = 18,684$)

Records screened ($n = 18,684$)

Records excluded ($n = 17,255$)

Full-text articles assessed for eligibility
($n = 1,429$)

Full text articles excluded, with reasons ($n = 1,423$)
Other Chinese Medicine interventions ($n = 1328$)
Did not meet inclusion criteria ($n = 63$)
Review article ($n = 26$)
Control includes CM ($n = 3$)
Other Chinese Medicine therapies ($n = 2$)
Duplicate literature ($n = 1$)

Non-controlled studies
($n = 5$)

Non-randomised controlled trials
($n = 0$)

Randomised controlled trials
($n = 1$)

Risk of Bias

The study was randomised and open label. Blinding of participants, personnel and outcome assessors was not performed and the study was at high risk of bias. Incomplete outcome data was at low risk of bias because there were no drop-outs. Selective outcome reporting was unclear because the study did not have a protocol. The overall methodological quality was low.

Cupping Therapy

Meta-analysis was not possible because there was only one study. Effective rate was the only reported outcome, defined by the Bronchial Asthma Guide.[3] It showed that cupping plus routine pharmacotherapy was better than routine pharmacotherapy alone (risk ratio 1.23; [1.07, 1.42]) (O1). The study did not mention if adverse events occurred.

Controlled Clinical Trials of Other Chinese Medicine Therapies

Non-randomised controlled trials were not found.

Non-controlled Clinical Studies of Other Chinese Medicine Therapies

Non-controlled studies evaluated cupping (two studies) (O2-O3), *tuina* 推拿 (two studies) (O4-O5), and *qigong* 气功 (one study) (O6). Lung *qi* deficiency was reported in one study that evaluated cupping (O3).

In one of the cupping studies, cups were applied to acupuncture points, EX-B1 *Dingchuan* 定喘 and BL13 *Feishu* 肺俞 and the other study did not report the method. In the *qigong* 气功 study, *yangsheng* style was performed. The two studies that evaluated *tuina* 推拿 did not report the method. One study reported that no adverse events occurred after *tuina* 推拿. The other four studies did not report if adverse events had occurred.

Summary of Other Chinese Medicine Clinical Evidence

Currently, there are a limited number of studies that evaluate other CM therapies for asthma. Therapies include cupping, *tuina* 推拿, and *qigong* 气功. In a randomised controlled trial, cupping improved effective rate. There were no non-randomised controlled clinical trials and only five non-controlled studies. Overall, there is not enough research to determine if other CM therapies are effective or safe for the treatment of asthma.

References

1. Sharma M, Taj. Tai Chi as an Alternative and Complementary Therapy for Patients With Asthma and Chronic Obstructive Pulmonary Disease: A Systematic Review. Evid Based Complement Alternat Med. 2013;**18**(3):209–15.
2. Cao H, Han M, Li X, Dong S, Wang Y, Xu Q, Liu S, J. Clinical research evidence of cupping therapy in China: a systematic literature review. BMC Complement Altern Med. 2010;**10**:70.
3. Prevention and treatment of asthma guideline. (1997) Chin J Tuberc Respir Dis, 20(5):261–267. [In Chinese: 支气管哮喘防治指南. 中华结核和呼吸杂志, 1997;**20**(5):261–267].

References to Included Other Chinese Medicine Therapies

Study No.	Reference
O1	陈国廉, 肖国民. 脏腑背俞排罐疗法治疗缓解期支气管哮喘的临床研究. 卫生职业教育. 2013,31(15):156–157,158
O2	冯军, 唐强, 陆岩. 于致顺教授应用刺络拔罐法临床治验举隅. 针灸临床杂志. 1995;(02):3.

(Continued)

(*Continued*)

Study No.	Reference
O3	Wang QR, Wang CS, Wang XJ. Medication with bricanyl supplemented by cupping in the treatment of 50 cases of asthma. *Int J Clin Acupunct* 1995;6(4):427–9.
O4	容斌 刘. 推拿治疗支气管哮喘 35 例. 陕西中医. 2005;26(12):1364–5.
O5	付强 苏, 杨永明, 张维,. 内科推拿在治疗哮喘各期中的临床应用. 按摩与康复医学. 2012;3(32):72–3.
O6	Reuther I, Aldridge D. Qigong Yangsheng as a complementary therapy in the management of asthma: a single-case appraisal. *J Alt Comp Med* 1998;4(2):173–83.

9

Clinical Evidence for Combination Therapies

OVERVIEW

Chinese medicine therapies can be combined to enhance treatment effects. Combination therapies are common in clinical practice and may include Chinese herbal medicine plus acupuncture, cupping, or another procedure. A comprehensive search of nine scientific databases identified more than 20,000 citations. These were reviewed against rigorous inclusion criteria and two randomised controlled trials were included for analysis. Treatments included oral Chinese herbal medicine combined with electroacupuncture and herbal wash combined with the use of plum-blossom needles.

Introduction

Combination therapies are defined as two or more Chinese medicine (CM) interventions administered together, such as herbal medicine with acupuncture or cupping with acupuncture. Included studies are indicated by a "C" followed by a number, e.g. (C1). The reference list for included studies can be found at the end of this chapter. Database searches found 28,153 citations, and among these, 18,684 were screened and 1,429 were subject to full-text review. Combinations of CM therapies for asthma have been evaluated in two randomised controlled trials (RCTs) that met the inclusion criteria (C1–C2) (Fig. 9.1).

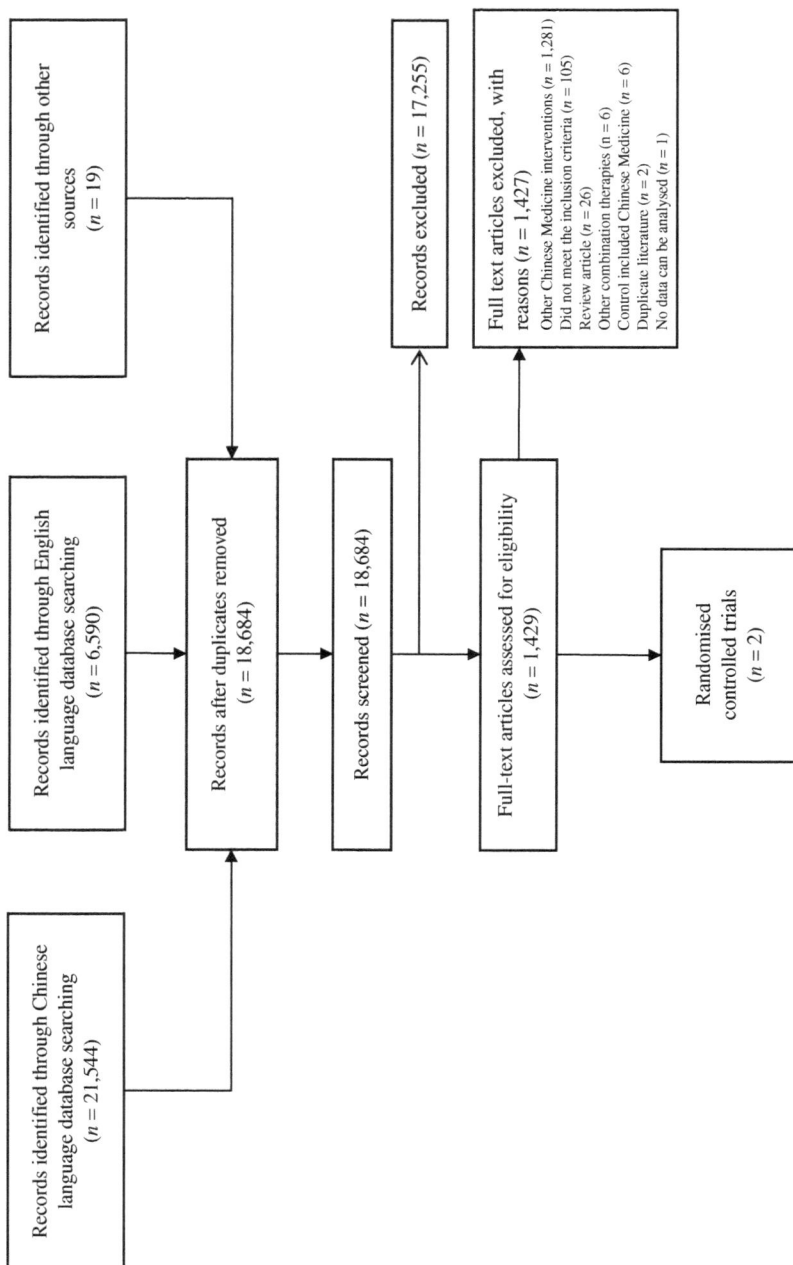

Figure 9.1 Flow chart of study selection process: combination therapies.

Characteristics of Clinical Studies of Combination Therapies

Oral Chinese herbal medicine (CHM) plus electroacupuncture was evaluated in one study and herbal wash plus plum-blossom needle was evaluated in the other study. Both studies compared a combination of CM therapies with pharmacotherapy to pharmacotherapy alone.

In total, 210 people participated in the studies and age ranged from 19 to 65 years. Treatment duration in the study that evaluated herbal wash plus plum-blossom needle was two weeks (C1) and the other study did not mention the treatment duration (C2). CM syndromes were not described in the studies.

Risk of Bias

Risk of bias was high because none of the studies reported either appropriate randomisation methods or allocation concealment. In addition, the participants and research personnel were not blinded. All participants completed the studies and therefore bias was low for incomplete outcome data. The studies did not have published protocols and thus present unclear risk of bias in terms of selective outcome reporting. The overall methodological quality of studies included in this section was low.

Chinese Herbal Medicine plus Electroacupuncture

One study evaluated formulae based on syndrome differentiation and electroacupuncture plus pharmacotherapy during acute exacerbations of asthma. Effective rate in terms of the Bronchial Asthma Guide did not improve (risk ratio 1.18 [0.99, 1.40]) (C2).

Herbal Wash plus Plum-blossom Needle

One study used a combination of herbal wash and plum-blossom needles over the back area plus pharmacotherapy for chronic asthma. The effective rate based on the Bronchial Asthma Guide was improved by 1.19 times that of pharmacotherapy alone [1.04, 1.37] (C1).

Summary of Evidence from Combination Therapies

Combination therapies were diverse and could not be pooled in the current meta-analysis. Included studies evaluated effective rate but not other asthma outcomes such as lung function. The studies did not report if adverse events occurred. Overall, studies evaluating combination CM therapies were limited in number. These studies provided some evidence that combination therapies can improve the total effective rate of treatment. However, results from the current research do not provide strong evidence to make specific recommendations for clinical practice.

References Included Combination Therapies Studies

Study No.	Reference
C1	石焱.三伏天中药液擦背治疗支气管哮喘 64 例临床观察. 浙江中医杂志. 2010,45(12):890
C2	白明.中西医结合治疗支气管哮喘 43 例. 河南中医. 2013,33(11): 1988–1989

10

Summary and Conclusions

OVERVIEW

Chinese medicine is commonly used to treat asthma. Over 300 clinical studies have evaluated the effects of Chinese medicine on adult asthma, including 333 assessing Chinese herbal medicine, 49 assessing acupuncture and related therapies, six assessing other Chinese medicine therapies, and two assessing combination therapies. This chapter provides a "whole evidence" analysis of Chinese medicine for the management of asthma.

Introduction

Chinese medicine (CM) therapies are increasingly used to treat asthma, and many clinical studies have been conducted in light of this growing trend. Control of symptoms is the main treatment goal and CM may offer beneficial effects for asthma. Evidence from clinical studies revealed promising benefits of Chinese herbal medicine (CHM), acupuncture, and various other CM therapies. This monograph utilizes a 'whole evidence' analysis to investigate CM for the management of asthma. Review of the classical literature identified a range of herbal medicines and acupuncture points which have been used to treat asthma. This has been supported by modern research from clinical studies which also revealed promising benefits of CHM and acupuncture. Our contemporary literature, which encompasses clinical guidelines and textbooks, thus recommends a broad range of CHM and acupuncture treatments for asthma.

Chinese Herbal Medicine

Evidence from classical literature reveals that CHM has been consistently used to treat asthma. Over time, the nomenclature has changed and the terms used to describe asthma have varied. However, herbal formulae and herbs, including *ban xia* 半夏, *gan cao* 甘草, *xing ren* 杏仁, and *ma huang* 麻黄, have been used for centuries to treat asthma symptoms. Modern treatment guidelines and textbooks based on classical literature outline the main syndromes and treatments and serve as a useful guide for clinical decision making. CHM has also been examined in more than 300 clinical trials and in experimental studies.

The common CM syndromes described in contemporary literature and clinical studies are categorised as excess and deficiency types of asthma. Syndromes include excess cold, heat, wind, phlegm, wheeze and/or Lung-Spleen *qi* deficiency, or Lung-Kidney deficiency. During acute exacerbations, pathogenic factors should be the primary focus of herbal medicine treatment, while deficiencies should be tonified during the stable stages of asthma.

In clinical studies, common formulae include *Xiao qing long tang* 小青龙汤, *Ding chuan tang* 定喘汤, and *She gan ma huang tang* 射干麻黄汤. Overall, the most common herbs for asthma include *ma huang* 麻黄, *gan cao* 甘草, *xing ren* 杏仁, and *ban xia* 半夏. Commonly used herbs in clinical trials have also been examined in experimental studies. These herbs affect biochemical pathways that control inflammation and airway hyperresponsiveness, which are the main physiological determinants of asthma. These herbs have also been identified and described in classical literature as well as contemporary asthma guidelines and textbooks (Table 10.1).

Findings from Chinese Herbal Medicine Clinical Trials

Findings from 246 randomised controlled trials (RCTs) suggest that CHM leads to clinically important improvements during chronic asthma and acute exacerbations of asthma.

Table 10.1   Summary of CHM Formulae

Formula Name	Evidence in Contemporary Literature	Evidence in Classical Literature (No. of Citations)	Evidence in Clinical Studies		
			RCTs (No. of Studies)	CCTs (No. of Studies)	Non-controlled Studies (No. of Studies)
She gan ma huang tang 射干麻黄汤	Yes	51	8	0	1
Ma xing shi gan tang 麻杏石甘汤	Yes	0	6	0	1
Huang long shu chuang tang 黄龙舒喘汤	Yes	0	0	0	0
San zi yang qin tang 三子养亲汤	Yes	1	3	0	1
Ping chuan gu ben tang 平喘固本汤	Yes	0	0	0	0
Hui yang ji jiu tang 回阳急救汤	Yes	0	0	0	0
Liu jun zi tang 六君子汤	Yes	10	1	1	0
Bu fei san plus jin shui liu jun jian 补肺散, 合金水六君煎	Yes	0	0	0	0
Xiao qing long tang 小青龙汤	No	25	13	0	3
Bu zhong yi qi tang 补中益气汤	No	0	4	0	1
Ding chuan tang 定喘汤	No	22	8	0	4

Abbreviations: CCTs, Controlled Clinical Trials; CHM, Chinese Herbal Medicine; RCTs, Randomised Controlled Trials.

Chronic Asthma

- A total of 124 RCTs evaluated chronic asthma.
- CHM compared with placebos improved asthma control, reduced exacerbation frequency, and reduced use of rescue medication

(i.e., salbutamol). Health-related quality of life (HR-QoL) and effective rate were not measured in the RCTs.

- CHM compared with pharmacotherapy improved lung function and effective rate. Asthma control, exacerbation frequency, use of rescue medication, and HR-QoL were not measured in the RCTs.
- CHM plus pharmacotherapy compared with pharmacotherapy alone improved lung function, asthma control, and effective rate, and also reduced exacerbation frequency and use of rescue medication. There was no documented improvement of HR-QoL from CHM.
- Study quality was moderate for placebo-controlled studies and low to very low quality for other studies. The main limitations of these studies were the lack of adequate blinding of participants, personnel, and outcome assessors, and considerable heterogeneity of data between studies.
- CHM was found to be well tolerated by people with chronic asthma.

Acute Exacerbations of Asthma

- A total of 122 RCTs evaluated acute exacerbations of asthma.
- CHM compared with placebo improved lung function. Asthma control, use of rescue medication, HR-QoL, and effective rate were not measured in the RCTs.
- CHM compared with pharmacotherapy did not improve lung function and effective rate. Asthma control, use of rescue medication, and HR-QoL were not measured in the RCTs.
- CHM plus pharmacotherapy compared with pharmacotherapy alone improved lung function and effective rate. Asthma control and use of rescue medication was not found to be improved by CHM plus pharmacotherapy. HR-QoL was not measured in the RCTs.
- Study quality was moderate for placebo-controlled studies and low to very low quality for other studies. The main limitations were

the lack of adequate blinding of participants, personnel, and outcome assessors, and considerable heterogeneity of data between studies.

• CHM was well tolerated by people with acute exacerbations of asthma.

Acupuncture and Related Therapies

Acupuncture and related therapies, such as needle acupuncture, moxibustion, laser acupuncture, electroacupuncture, ultrasonic leading, acupoint magnet therapy, acupressure, ear acupressure, hot compress acupressure, scalp acupuncture, and transcutaneous electrical nerve stimulation (TENS) acupuncture have been assessed in clinical trials. Acupuncture points on the Conception Vessel, Stomach, and Kidney were most commonly mentioned in classical literature citations, and in contemporary literature these meridians are still important for treating asthma. Points such as CV22 *Tiantu* 天突, CV17 *Danzhong* 膻中, and ST36 *Zusanli* 足三里 were often mentioned in the classical literature and are still used today, with the exception of EX-B1 *Dingchuan* 定喘 which is commonly used today but was seldom mentioned in the classical literature.

Acupuncture therapies have expanded over recent times and therapies such as acupressure, scalp acupuncture, laser acupuncture, and acupoint magnet therapy have been evaluated in clinical studies. However, the main acupuncture therapies recommended in clinical practice have also been described in classical literature as well as contemporary asthma guidelines and textbooks (Table 10.2). In contemporary literature, syndromes and symptoms are used to guide acupuncture point selection, although many clinical trials do not report CM syndromes. Lung, Spleen, and Kidney *qi* deficiency was the most frequently reported syndrome followed by phlegm-heat or phlegm-cold. The most frequently used acupuncture point was BL13 *Feishu* 肺俞. Other common points included EX-B1 *Dingchuan* 定喘, CV22 *Tiantu* 天突, and GV14 *Dazhui* 大椎.

Table 10.2   Summary of Acupuncture and Related Therapies

Acupuncture Intervention	Evidence in Contemporary Literature	Evidence in Classical Literature (No. of Citations)	Evidence in Clinical Studies		
			RCTs (No. of Studies)	CCTs[#] (No. of Studies)	Non-controlled Studies[#] (No. of Studies)
Acupuncture	Yes	16	14	0	4
Moxibustion	Yes	34	14	0	4
Electroacupuncture or TENS	No	0	2	0	1
Acupressure	No	2	1	0	0
Laser acupuncture	No	0	1	0	2
Acupoint magnet therapy	No	0	1	0	0
Ear acupressure	No	0	1	0	0
Scalp acupuncture	No	0	1	0	0
BL13 Feishu 肺俞	Yes	15	21	0	9
EX-B1 Dingchuan 定喘	Yes	0	12	0	6
ST36 Zusanli 足三里	Yes	21	8	0	4
CV22 Tiantu 天突	Yes	35	6	0	3
BL20 Pishu 脾俞	No	0	5	0	3
CV17 Danzhong 膻中	Yes	20	7	0	1
GV14 Dazhui 大椎	Yes	0	5	0	3
LI4 Hegu 合谷	No	0	6	0	2
LU6 Kongzui 孔最	No	0	8	0	0
ST40 Fenglong 丰隆	Yes	4	4	0	4

Abbreviations: CCTs, Controlled Clinical Trials; RCTs, Randomised Controlled Trials.
[#]There were no CCT studies.

Findings from Clinical Trials of Acupuncture and Related Therapies

Findings from 36 RCTs suggest that acupuncture improves clinically important outcomes during chronic asthma and acute exacerbations of asthma.

Acupuncture

- A total of 14 studies evaluated acupuncture.
- Compared with sham acupuncture, lung function was improved. Use of rescue medication and effective rate were not improved in the acupuncture groups compared with sham acupuncture or pharmacotherapy.
- Acupuncture combined with pharmacotherapy compared to pharmacotherapy alone improved HR-QoL and effective rate. Lung function, asthma control, and use of rescue medication were not measured.
- Study quality was moderate for sham-controlled studies and low for other studies. The main limitations were the lack of adequate blinding of participants, personnel, and outcome assessors, and small sample sizes.
- Acupuncture was well tolerated by people with asthma.

Moxibustion

- A total of 14 studies evaluated moxibustion.
- Moxibustion compared with pharmacotherapy improved lung function but not asthma control or effective rate.
- Study quality was low due to lack of blinding of adequate blinding of participants, personnel, and outcome assessors, and small sample sizes.
- Moxibustion did not produce any significant adverse effects.

Other related therapies such as electroacupuncture, acupressure, acupoint magnet therapy, laser acupuncture, and scalp acupuncture were evaluated in a very small number of studies. Some results were positive, but quality was limited by lack of adequate blinding of participants, personnel, and outcome assessors, as well as small sample sizes. Most studies did not report if adverse events occurred.

Other Chinese Medicine Therapies

Six clinical trials evaluated other CM therapies including cupping, *tuina* 推拿, and *qigong* 气功 for asthma. Contemporary guidelines

Table 10.3 Summary of Other CM Therapies

Other Therapies	Evidence in Contemporary Literature	Evidence in Classical Literature (No. of Citations)	Evidence in Clinical Studies		
			RCTs (No. of Studies)	CCTs (No. of Studies)	Non-controlled Studies (No. of Studies)
Qigong 气功	Yes	0	0	0	1
Cupping	No	2	1	0	2
Tuina 推拿	No	0	0	0	2

Abbreviations: CCTs, Controlled Clinical Trials; CM, Chinese Medicine; RCTs, Randomised Controlled Trials.

and classical literature citations also recommend *qigong* 气功 to maintain physical strength and resistance (Table 10.3).

Only one RCT could be analysed and it showed that cupping plus pharmacotherapy was better than pharmacotherapy alone in terms of effective rate. Other outcomes such as lung function and asthma control were not measured, and adverse events were not mentioned.

Implications for Practice

The classical literature shows that many citations are broadly consistent with asthma as it is known today. The results indicate that most formulae, herbs, and acupuncture points are similar in modern clinical practice. These interventions may guide further practice through their exploration in clinical and experimental research. Findings from randomised controlled trials suggest that CHM leads to clinically important improvements including lung function and effective rate during acute exacerbations and chronic asthma. CHM was well tolerated for people with asthma.

Acupuncture and related therapies have been cited in classical literature and are commonly used in modern clinical practice. Some acupuncture points are used in both ancient and modern times. Acupuncture was overall well tolerated.

Results from other CM therapies, such as cupping, *tuina* 推拿, and *qigong* 气功, are somewhat encouraging, but the confidence of these results are limited as only a small number of studies have been conducted thus far. These preliminary findings suggest that these therapies may be used by asthma patients and do not appear to be harmful, but more studies need to be done. Combination therapies have also been studied in a small number of RCTs and overall there is a lack of evidence for combination therapies.

Implications for Research

Clinical trials of CM therapies have increased in recent decades. This trend reflects the desire for evidence-based medicine and the use of science and technology to validate medical practices and their effects. The information gained from research on CM therapies for asthma suggests some important possible future research directions.

The methodological quality of the clinical trials of asthma is moderate or low. Rigorous study designs are needed to evaluate these promising interventions and produce better quality evidence. Therefore, studies should include properly validated outcomes. Effective rate can be measured using various validated criteria, including the Traditional Chinese Medicine (TCM) Syndrome Diagnostic efficacy standards, CM clinical research guidelines, and Bronchial Asthma Guide. Despite the availability of established guidelines, effective rate is not a validated outcome measure for asthma and results can be inconsistent and unreliable. In addition, clinical trial protocols should be published and made available for reference. Research reports should follow the CONSORT statement with reference to the extension for herbal medicine[1,2] and STRICTA for clinical trials of acupuncture.[3]

Diversity was seen in the range of CM therapies reflecting the nature of CM clinical practice. Future research should focus on the most promising findings identified and investigate therapies that can be widely used. Standardised herbal formula, specific sets of acupuncture points, and combination CM therapies are suitable areas for future research.

References

1. Schulz KF, Altman DG, Moher D. CONSORT 2010 statement: Updated guidelines for reporting parallel group randomized trials. *Ann Intern Med*. 2010;**152**(11):726–32.
2. Gagnier JJ, Boon H, Rochon P, Moher D, Barnes J, Bombardier C. Reporting randomized, controlled trials of herbal interventions: An elaborated CONSORT statement. *Ann Intern Med*. 2006;**144**(5): 364–7.
3. MacPherson H, White A, Cummings M, Jobst K, Rose K, Niemtzow, R. Standards for reporting interventions in controlled trials of acupuncture: The STRICTA recommendations. *Complement Ther Med*. 2001;**9**(4):246–9.

Glossary

Terms	Acronym	Definition	Reference
95% Confidence Interval	95% CI	A measure of the uncertainty around the main finding of a statistical analysis. Estimates of unknown quantities, such as the odds ratio comparing an experimental intervention with a control, are usually presented as a point estimate and a 95% confidence interval. This means that if someone were to keep repeating a study in other samples from the same population, 95% of the confidence intervals from those studies would contain the true value of the unknown quantity. Alternatives to 95%, such as 90% and 99% confidence intervals, are sometimes used. Wider intervals indicate lower precision; narrow intervals, greater precision.	http://handbook.cochrane.org/
Acupressure	—	Application of pressure on acupuncture points.	—
Acupuncture	—	The insertion of needles into humans or animals for remedial purposes or its methods.	WHO International Standard Terminologies of Traditional Medicine in the Western Pacific Region. World Health Organisation; 2007.
Allied and Complementary Medicine Database	AMED	Alternative medicine bibliographic database	https://www.ebscohost.com/academic/AMED-The-Allied-and-Complementary-Medicine-Database

American Thoracic Society	ATS	Medical association dedicated to advancing clinical and scientific understanding of pulmonary diseases, critical illnesses and sleep-related breathing disorders.	http://www.thoracic.org/
Asthma Control Test	ACT	A patient self-administered tool for identifying those with poorly controlled asthma: 5 items, with 4-week recall (symptoms and daily functioning).	Nathan RA, Sorkness CA, Kosinski M, Schatz M, Li JT, Marcus P, Murray JJ, Pendergraft TB. Development of the asthma control test: A survey for assessing asthma control. J Allergy Clin Immunol 2004 (113): 59–65.
Asthma Quality of Life Questionnaire	AQLQ	A disease-specific health-related quality of life instrument that assess both physical and emotional impact of disease: 32 items with 2-week recall.	Juniper EF, Guyatt GH, Willan A, Griffith LE. Determining a minimal important change in a disease-specific quality of life questionnaire. J Clin Epidemiol 1994; 47(1): 81–87.
Australian New Zealand Clinical Trial Registry	ANZCTR	Australian clinical trial registry	http://www.anzctr.org.au/
China National Knowledge Infrastructure	CNKI	Chinese language bibliographic database	http://www.cnki.net/

(Continued)

Terms	Acronym	Definition	Reference
Chinese Biomedical Literature Database	CBM	Chinese language bibliographic database	https://cbmwww.imicams.ac.cn
Chinese Clinical Trial Registry	ChiCTR	Chinese clinical trial registry	http://www.chictr.org
Chinese Herbal Medicine	CHM	Chinese herbal medicine	—
Chinese Medicine	CM	—	—
Chongqing VIP Information Company	CQVIP	Chinese language bibliographic database	http://www.cqvip.com/
ClinicalTrials.gov	—	Clinical trial registry	https://www.clinicaltrials.gov/
Cochrane Central Register of Controlled Trials	CENTRAL	Bibliographic database that provides a highly concentrated source of reports of controlled trials.	http://community.cochrane.org/editorial-and-publishing-policy-resource/cochrane-central-register-controlled-trials-central
Combination Therapies	—	Two or more Chinese medicines from different therapy groups (e.g., Chinese herbal medicine, acupuncture therapies, or other Chinese medicine therapies) administered together.	—
Convention on International Trade in Endangered Species of Wild Fauna and Flora	CITES	—	https://www.cites.org/eng/disc/text.php

Term	Abbreviation	Definition	Source
Cumulative Index of Nursing and Allied Health Literature	CINAHL	Bibliographic database	https://www.ebscohost.com/nursing/about
Cupping therapy	—	Suction by using a vaccumised cup or jar.	WHO International Standard Terminologies of Traditional Medicine in the Western Pacific Region. World Health Organisation; 2007.
Effect size	—	A generic term for the estimate of effect of treatment for a study.	http://handbook.cochrane.org/
Effective rate	—	A measure of the proportion of participants who achieved an improvement, as outlined in the Clinical evidence section.	—
Electroacupuncture	—	Electric stimulation of the needle following insertion.	WHO International Standard Terminologies of Traditional Medicine in the Western Pacific Region. World Health Organisation; 2007.
EU Clinical Trials Register	EU-CTR	European clinical trial registry	https://www.clinicaltrialsregister.eu/
Excerpta Medica Database	Embase	Bibliographic database	http://www.elsevier.com/solutions/embase

(Continued)

Terms	Acronym	Definition	Reference
Forced Expiratory Volume in One Second	FEV_1	Volume of air exhaled during one second, usually measured in litres or percent.	Brooker C. Mosby's dictionary of medicine, nursing and health professions. Elsevier: United Kingdom; 2010.
Forced Vital Capacity	FVC	The maximum gas volume that can be expelled from the lungs in a forced expiration.	Brooker C. Mosby's dictionary of medicine, nursing and health professions. Elsevier: United Kingdom; 2010.
Global Initiative for Asthma	GINA	—	http://www.ginasthma.org/
Grading of Recommendations Assessment, Development, and Evaluation	GRADE	Approach used to grade quality of evidence and strength of recommendations.	http://www.gradeworkinggroup.org/
Health-related Quality of Life	HR-QoL	A conceptual or operational measurement that is commonly used in the health care setting as a means to assess the impact of disease on the person.	Brooker C. Mosby's dictionary of medicine, nursing and health professions. Elsevier: United Kingdom; 2010.
Heterogeneity	—	Used in a general sense to describe the variation in, or diversity of, participants, interventions, and measurement of outcomes across a set of studies, or the variation in internal validity of those studies.	http://handbook.cochrane.org/

Term		Definition	Source
		When used specifically as statistical heterogeneity, heterogeneity describes the degree of variation in the effect estimates from a set of studies. Also used to indicate the presence of variability among studies beyond the amount expected due solely to chance.	http://handbook.cochrane.org/
Homogeneity	—	Used in a general sense to mean that the participants, interventions, and measurement of outcomes are similar across a set of studies. Used specifically to describe the effect estimates from a set of studies where they do not vary more than would be expected by chance.	
I^2	—	A measure of heterogeneity, which indicates the percentage of variance in a meta-analysis.	http://handbook.cochrane.org/
Inhaled Corticosteroids	ICS	Glucocorticoids designed to be inhaled for treatment of the respiratory tract and lungs.	
Integrative Medicine	—	Chinese herbal medicine combined with pharmacotherapy or other conventional therapy.	
Long-acting Beta2 Agonists	LABA	Class of drugs that act on the beta2-adrenergic receptor causing smooth muscle relaxation. Duration of action is approximately 12 hours.	

(Continued)

Terms	Acronym	Definition	Reference
Mean Difference	MD	In meta-analysis, mean difference is a method used to combine measures on continuous scales where the mean, standard deviation, and sample size in each group are known. The weight given to the difference in means from each study (e.g., how much influence each study has on the overall results of the meta-analysis) is determined by the precision of its estimate of effect. Mathematically, this is equal to the inverse of the variance. This method assumes that all of the trials have measured the outcome on the same scale.	http://handbook.cochrane.org/
Meta-analysis	—	The use of statistical techniques in a systematic review to integrate the results of included studies. Sometimes misused as a synonym for systematic reviews, where the review includes a meta-analysis.	—
Moxibustion	—	A therapeutic procedure involving ignited material (usually moxa) to apply heat to certain points or areas of the body surface for curing disease through regulation of the function of meridians/channels and visceral organs.	WHO International Standard Terminologies of Traditional Medicine in the Western Pacific Region. World Health Organisation; 2007.

Term	Abbreviation	Definition	URL
Non-controlled Studies	—	Observations made on individuals, usually receiving the same intervention, before and after an intervention but with no control group.	http://handbook.cochrane.org/
Controlled Clinical Trials	CCT	An experimental study in which people are allocated to different interventions using methods that are not random.	http://handbook.cochrane.org/
Other Chinese Medicine Therapies	—	Other Chinese medicine therapies include all traditional therapies except Chinese herbal medicine and acupuncture, such as *tai chi, qigong, tuina,* and cupping.	
Peak Expiratory Flow	PEF	Assesses a person's degree of obstruction in the airways by measuring the maximum speed of expiration with a peak flow meter. Also called peak expiratory flow rate (PEFR).	
PubMed	PubMed	Bibliographic database	http://www.ncbi.nlm.nih.gov/pubmed
Qigong 气功	—	Physical exercises and breathing techniques.	—
Randomised Controlled Trial	RCT	Clinical trial that uses a random method to allocate participants to treatment and control groups.	—
Risk of Bias	—	Assessment of clinical trials to indicate if results may overestimate or underestimate the true effect because of bias in study design or reporting.	http://handbook.cochrane.org/

(Continued)

Terms	Acronym	Definition	Reference
Risk Ratio	RR	The ratio of risks in two groups. In intervention studies, it is the ratio of the risk in the intervention group to the risk in the control group. A risk ratio of one indicates no difference between comparison groups. For undesirable outcomes, a risk ratio that is less than one indicates that the intervention was effective in reducing the risk of that outcome.	http://handbook.cochrane.org/
Short-acting Beta2 Agonists	SABA	Class of drugs that act on the beta2-adrenergic receptor causing smooth muscle relaxation. Duration of action is 4–6 hours.	
Summary of Findings	—	Presentation of results and rating the quality of evidence based on the GRADE approach.	http://www. gradeworkinggroup.org/
Tai chi 推拿	—	Physical exercises and breathing techniques.	—
Transcutaneous electrical nerve stimulation	TENS	Application of transdermal electrical current to acupuncture points via conducting pads.	—
Tuina 推拿	—	A form of Chinese massage, which includes rubbing, kneading, or percussion of the soft tissues and joints of the body with the hands, usually performed by one person on another, especially to relieve tension or pain.	WHO International Standard Terminologies of Traditional Medicine in the Western Pacific Region. World Health Organisation; 2007.
Tumour Necrosis Factor-Alpha	TNF-α	A cytokine that is toxic to cancer cells and activates other leukocytes. It causes profound metabolic effects that include inflammatory responses, pyrexia, and weight loss leading to cachexia.	Brooker C. Mosby's dictionary of medicine, nursing and health professions. Elsevier: United Kingdom; 2010.

Term	Abbreviation	Description	Reference
Wangfang Database	Wanfang	Chinese language bibliographic database	www.wanfangdata.com
World Health Organisation	WHO	WHO is the directing and coordinating authority for health within the United Nations system. It is responsible for providing leadership on global health matters, shaping the health research agenda, setting norms and standards, articulating evidence-based policy options, providing technical support to countries, and monitoring and assessing health trends.	http://www.who.int/about/en/
Zhong Hua Yi Dian 中华医典	ZHYD	Also known as the *Encyclopaedia of Traditional Chinese Medicine*, the ZHYD is a comprehensive series of electronic books put together by the Hunan Electronic and Audio-visual Publishing House. It is the largest collection of Chinese electronic books and includes major Chinese ancient works, many of which are from rare manuscripts and are the only existing copies. These books cover the period from ancient times up to the period of the Republic of China (1911–1948).	Hu R, editor. Zhong Hua Yi Dian [Encyclopaedia of Traditional Chinese Medicine]. 4th ed. Chengsha: Hunan Electronic and Audio-Visual Publishing House; 2000.
Zhong Yi Fang Ji Da Ci Dian 中医方剂大辞典	ZYFJDCD	Compendium of Chinese herbal formulae with over 96,592 entries derived from classical Chinese books. The Nanjing Chinese Medicine Institute compiled the ZYFJDCD and first published it in 1993.	

Index

www.ingramcontent.com/pod-product-compliance
Lightning Source LLC
Chambersburg PA
CBHW050600190326
41458CB00007B/2114